W9-AFU-255

The

AUTISM BOOK

THE
AUTISM BOOK

· ·

Answers to Your Most Pressing Questions

· ·

S. Jhoanna Robledo
and
Dawn Ham-Kucharski

Foreword by Richard Solomon, M.D.

AVERY
a member of
Penguin Group (USA) Inc.
New York

Published by the Penguin Group

Penguin Group (USA) Inc., 375 Hudson Street, New York, New York 10014, USA ·
Penguin Group (Canada), 10 Alcorn Avenue, Toronto, Ontario M4V 3B2, Canada (a division
of Pearson Penguin Canada Inc.) · Penguin Books Ltd, 80 Strand, London WC2R 0RL,
England · Penguin Ireland, 25 St Stephen's Green, Dublin 2, Ireland (a division of Penguin
Books Ltd) · Penguin Group (Australia), 250 Camberwell Road, Victoria 3124,
Australia (a division of Pearson Australia Group Pty Ltd) · Penguin Books India Pvt Ltd,
11 Community Centre, Panchsheel Park, New Delhi–110 017, India · Penguin Group (NZ),
Cnr Airborne and Rosedale Roads, Albany, Auckland 1310, New Zealand (a division of Pearson
New Zealand Ltd) · Penguin Books (South Africa) (Pty) Ltd, 24 Sturdee Avenue, Rosebank,
Johannesburg 2196, South Africa · Penguin Books Ltd, Registered Offices:
80 Strand, London WC2R 0RL, England

Copyright © 2005 by S. Jhoanna Robledo and Dawn Ham-Kucharski
All rights reserved. No part of this book may be reproduced, scanned, or distributed
in any printed or electronic form without permission. Please do not participate
in or encourage piracy of copyrighted materials in violation
of the authors' rights. Purchase only authorized editions.
Published simultaneously in Canada

Library of Congress Cataloging-in-Publication Data

Robledo, S. Jhoanna.
The autism book : answers to your most pressing questions /
S. Jhoanna Robledo and Dawn Ham-Kucharski.
p.   cm.
Includes bibliographical references and index.
ISBN 1-58333-224-3
1. Autism in children—Miscellanea.   I. Ham-Kucharski, Dawn.   II. Title.
RJ506.A9R625   2005   2004062819
618.92'85882—dc22

Printed in the United States of America
1   3   5   7   9   10   8   6   4   2

Neither the authors nor the publisher is engaged in rendering professional advice or services to the individual reader. The ideas, procedures, and suggestions in this book are not intended as a substitute for consulting a physician. All matters regarding health require medical supervision. Neither the authors nor the publisher shall be liable or responsible for any loss, injury, or damage allegedly arising from any information or suggestion in this book. The opinions expressed in this book represent the personal views of the authors and not of the publisher.

While the authors have made every effort to provide accurate telephone numbers and Internet addresses at the time of publication, neither the publisher nor the authors assume any responsibility for errors or for changes that occur after publication.

Most Avery books are available at special quantity discounts for bulk purchase for sales promotions, premiums, fund-raising, and educational needs. Special books or book excerpts also can be created to fit specific needs. For details, write Penguin Group (USA) Inc. Special Markets, 375 Hudson Street, New York, NY 10014.

Acknowledgments

We would like to thank our immediate and extended families and friends—especially Dave, Jackie, Ann, Paolo, and Lee—for supporting us through this entire process, from the moment we concocted the idea to its fruition. Specifically, we extend our gratitude to:

Our agent, Dan Bial, and editor, Kristen Jennings, for investing their time and energies into what may at first have appeared to be a quixotic project;

The grandparents, mothers, fathers, and siblings of autistic children who helped us hone the purpose, message, and content of the book;

The autism experts (teachers, therapists, and doctors), most notably Dr. Richard Solomon, who carved out time from their busy schedules to respond to the numerous questions we had about the condition;

Our husbands, Rich and Will, for being such doting fathers, encouraging partners, and our best friends;

Our parents, Jim (whom Alex believes is a star in the sky watching out for him), and Dorothy and Jeannie and Vincent, for raising us to believe that no goal is ever out of reach and for being so devoted to our children. Dorothy, especially, has been instrumental in the success of her grandson,

Alex, from whom she learns about, and shares with every day, the wonders of life;

Our grandparents, especially Verna (Alex's other star) and Quiller Kitto and Benedicto "Daddy" Celino, who inspired us to work on this meaningful project and forge on when all we had was a kernel of an idea;

Our children, who remind us every day of what's important and what's real—we are privileged to be able to watch you grow and learn about life.

This book is dedicated to Alex, Dawn's beautiful son, who teaches everyone who takes the time to get to know him how to see the world from his unique perspective. You are your mother's gift, her light and love, and an inspiration to children and adults on and off the spectrum.

And to children living with autism everywhere . . . you are all incredible.

Contents

Foreword

As a developmental and behavioral pediatrician who has, during the last fifteen years, treated well over a thousand children with autism, I know that when I make the heartrending diagnosis of "autistic spectrum disorder," I am sending a child's family down a long road that will be filled with questions. In this important book, Dawn Ham-Kucharski and S. Jhoanna Robledo accompany families down that road and patiently answer the pressing questions that families ask when confronted with the challenge of raising a young child with autism.

Dawn and her husband, Rich, are parents of Alex who, when I first met him and diagnosed his condition, was at the age of two locked into the wordless, self-isolating, repetitive world of autism. Now, at age six Alex is a delightful, talkative, charming, and successful student in a first-grade public school and special education class. Dawn's is a family that has walked the walk and, with the help of her close friend, Jhoanna, a seasoned medical writer, is talking the talk. All the basic questions are answered in this book, from *What is autism?* to *What types of treatments work for children with autism?* But even the hardest, most difficult questions that parents ask—*How do I handle negative comments from my relatives?* or *Why did this happen to us?*—are raised and explored. Sometimes there is no "right" answer. Nevertheless it is reassuring to know that the right questions can be asked.

And more families are asking questions because so many more young children, ages eighteen months to six years, are being identified with autistic spectrum disorders. The prevalence of autism is increasing at such an alarming rate (15 percent per year every year for the last twenty years in Michigan!) that the U.S. Centers for Disease Control and Prevention has called it an "epidemic." One of every 150 children has an autistic spectrum disorder. More than 1.5 million are affected, and autism is seemingly on the rise. In this book, read answers to the questions: *Is there an epidemic of autism?* or *Do vaccines cause autism?* or *Is autism hereditary?*

One thing we know for sure is that cold, "refrigerator" parents do not cause autism. Parents are not to blame. Autism is a neurological condition that causes the brain to divide into separate neuronal pathways. This disintegration of neurons leads to a fragmented worldview from which the child with autism looks at our most complex cultural accomplishments— language and social interactions—as alien and frightening. It is no wonder that these children want to stay in their comfort zones. So many important questions arise in parents' minds: *What does it mean when a child perseverates?* and *Why do children with autism perseverate on doors, lights, locks, wheels, etc.?* Understanding how a child with autism thinks is the first step toward helping him.

The Autism Book moves systematically from defining the diagnosis and listing known causes to describing the varied manifestations of this multifaceted condition. Then, based on hard-won experience, the authors closely and accurately follow the arc of parents' initial emotional reactions—*Will our lives ever be the same?* or *Where can I find other parents like me?*—to help them gain the emotional momentum they will need to provide the demanding interventions that young children with autism require. The authors rightly dispel old beliefs about autism being untreatable and they give families true reason to hope. But intervention, to be most successful, should start at the earliest possible moment. This book focuses on the importance of early intervention. The National Research Council in 2001 set out a standard, based both on research and sound clinical experience, for appropriate interventions that are effective for young children with autistic spectrum disorders. Most children with autism can be helped to make substantial and often dramatic gains in language and social skills when provided with appropriate amounts and types of early intervention. *Is there a cure for autism? What are the most common traditional therapies? What is ABA? What is Floortime? What is sensory integration therapy? What are my child's educational options?* These are questions every parent must know the answers to. Even questions about the various supportive and non-traditional therapies are fully described.

After parents have learned about and begun providing sound interventions, relentless, difficult questions persist: *My child seems to be improving with his therapy. Does this mean the worst is behind us?* Or *How do I explain autism to my child's brother/sister? How do I appropriately discipline my child?* And then there are the hardest questions of all, the ones that can never be answered by science: *My marriage has suffered from the challenges of raising an autistic child. How can we get help?* And the most emotionally devastating question: *What if, despite interventions, my child never gets any better?* This is where experience must supersede knowledge. For science, this is where the sidewalk ends. Dealing with family parenting and sibling issues, getting out and about, dealing with schools, facing worries—on these questions, sound research is only just beginning. We must rely on experience and learn to trust the guidance of shared wisdom.

Raising questions is one thing; answering them is another. As a physician who has spent all of his adult life in academia, I am steeped in scientific tradition. As I read this book's answers, I asked my own critical questions: Was the information thorough? Accurate? Well researched? Honest? Balanced when dealing with controversial issues? To each of these questions I can confidently say, Yes! I would also add that it is extremely well written. The authors have done a remarkably thorough job of bringing to parents (and professionals) the latest in scientific research on the topic of autism. As a clinician I know that science and research are not everything families need. They need caring, compassion, guidance, and wise counsel.

And the advice given here is caring, compassionate, and wise not only because it is based on Dawn's personal experience but because it is drawn from the broad experience of other parents all traveling the same road. Dawn is intimately involved and connected with the autism community of families and professionals and she is a leader within these communities.

Because of its intelligence and heart, I plan to recommend this book as the first book of answers any family should read as it takes that first step down this long road of questions.

Richard Solomon, M.D.
Medical director, the Ann Arbor Center for Development and Behavioral Pediatrics; adjunct clinical associate professor, University of Michigan; and director of the PLAY (Play and Language for Autistic Youngsters) Project

Introduction

Sometimes we choose to champion a cause because its mission speaks to us in ways that surprise us, encouraging us to imagine what it's like for others to suffer enormous challenges. But sometimes a cause simply chooses us.

When co-author Dawn Ham-Kucharski found out she was pregnant two years after my first child, Nina, was born, we celebrated with a vengeance. Best friends since graduate school, we were like sisters and welcomed each other's good news as if it were our own. Dawn, who lived in Michigan, looked forward to swapping baby tips with me in San Francisco, where I happened to be working at the time as a reporter and editor for a pregnancy, baby health, and parenting Web site. But in her thirty-second week of pregnancy, Dawn's health took a turn for the worse and she gave birth to a son, Alex, prematurely. When he was given the green light to go home weeks later, however, both Dawn and her family thought the worst was behind them.

When Alex was twenty-six months of age, however, Dawn, her husband, Rich, and her mother, Dorothy (who was always on hand to help with Alex), soon discovered there were more challenges to overcome.

They were well aware that Alex's temperament was different from that of most babies. Often described as an "easy child," he hardly made sounds or spoke, liked to stare at ceiling fans for hours, and never seemed to need or want his parents' attention. Dawn commiserated with me by phone about his unusual behavior, asking me to look up the latest research on a few developmental questions she had. But when Dawn took Alex to see the doctor, no one expected the diagnosis that was finally given them: Alex had "moderate to severe" autism.

The months and years that followed became a blur of doctors' visits, therapy sessions, psychological evaluations, and teacher meetings. Every time a new decision needed to be made, Dawn came up with even more questions to ask. Answers came few and far between, and I did my best to help Dawn find relevant and accurate information about everything from interventions to tips on how to handle the not always well-meaning comments from strangers.

One day in 2003, sympathetic to Dawn's frustrations over yet another complication, I asked, "Dawn, isn't there a book out there that can guide you through this whole process?" Dawn's reply stayed with me for weeks: "If there was a book that actually gave me straightforward answers, I would've bought it by now." At that time, I was writing freelance pieces for magazines and Web sites about health and nutrition and grieving the death of a beloved grandfather, who had always advised me to make my work purposeful. Thinking about the lack of information that must be available to countless parents out there, I offered a suggestion: Perhaps Dawn and I could team up to create a guide that would help parents just like Dawn. And so this book was born.

We don't purport to know everything there is to know about autism, but we've certainly done our best—with the help of the doctors, researchers, medical journals and studies, therapists, educational experts, and parents of autistic children we consulted for this project—to make this publication an accurate, comprehensive, friendly, and (we hope) supportive companion from the moment your child receives the diagnosis. These days, you don't have to muddle through the muck of information Dawn and her family had to sift through to get the help you and your child need now. Although there's room for improvement, many services are now available for children along the spectrum so they can have the best possible chance at living a fulfilling and joyful life. And although science still has a way to go before finding a cause, let alone a cure, now, more than ever, there's reason to hope for a bright future.

—S. Jhoanna Robledo and Dawn Ham-Kucharski

1.

DIAGNOSIS

. . . .

How do you know if your child is truly different from others? And in what way? In this chapter, you will find out what a diagnosis of autism means, how doctors know a child has it, and what lies before you in the months ahead.

What is autism?

Autism is a neurological disorder that usually manifests itself early in the toddler years. It hampers a child's ability to learn how to communicate, interact with others socially, and indulge in imaginative play. Classified officially as a pervasive developmental disorder (PDD), autism inhibits a child's development. For decades, autism has proven a challenge to scientists, who have come to understand just how complex it truly is. Although we know much more about it now than we did decades ago when doctors, led by child development expert Bruno Bettelheim, thought autism was caused by "refrigerator moms" who were distant or uncaring, the disorder is, in many ways, still a mystery. But autism is a puzzle that's chiseled at every day, so that at some time in the near future, we may have answers to its most vexing questions.

The term "autism" was first used in 1912 by scientist Eugene Bleuler, who also coined the term "schizophrenia," to describe a state of disassociation. But the first mention of autism as a disorder appeared in Baltimore doctor Leo Kanner's 1943 paper, "Autistic Disturbances of Affective Contact," which described his observations of children who exhibited symptoms that at the time were considered indicative of mental or emotional handicaps. A year later, Viennese doctor Hans Asperger wrote about a condition with symptoms strikingly comparable to those described by Kanner, and which was later termed Asperger's Syndrome, a type of autism.

Decades later, Bettelheim's theories about refrigerator moms were replaced by those of the less-accusatory Bernard Rimland, who discovered a biological root to the disorder. Today, scientists know that autism has nothing to do with how mothers treat their children and have traced the disorder to a genetic mutation in some of the body's chromosomes.

Over the years, as diagnostic criteria and procedures have improved, pediatricians, healthcare providers, and educators have gotten better at identifying children with autism. No wonder the disorder seems to be everywhere these days; stories about it routinely appear in both print and broadcast media, and nonprofit organizations devoted to advocacy and research have grown and expanded their outreach.

But for many families, autism is much more than merely a diagnosis. The clinical description fails to capture the grief and sorrow it elicits. Families with children who receive the diagnosis often feel as if their lives have been upended completely; to cope, they sometimes have to rethink their approach to parenting in everything from diet to education. They have to topple old expectations and build new ones, even as they scramble to find educational and therapeutic approaches that will give their children a chance to learn, grow, and be healthy. In short, they have to start from scratch.

Yet, while the learning curve may be steep, many families find that once they've assembled a support system that includes healthcare providers, relatives, teachers, therapists, and friends, they're able to recover their footing and steadily make progress, giving hope to others who may just be starting the long and sometimes discouraging journey to equilibrium.

How common is autism?

It's a lot more common than you may think. According to the Centers for Disease Control and Prevention, anywhere from 2 to 6 per 1,000 people are diagnosed with the disorder; the Autism Society of America pins it at about 1 in 250, which represents an estimated total of 1.5 million children and adults. The organization estimates that every day, fifty families in America discover that their child has autism. Many more children have some of the critical symptoms of autism, but not all. Thousands more languish on their own, still waiting to be diagnosed.

Is there an epidemic of autism?

The jury's still out on this one. Some experts say the numbers—which seem to be increasing every year at an alarming rate—point to a growing problem, but they fall short of actually calling the trend an epidemic. Still, a small number of experts have gone ahead and labeled it as such. The root of the discrepancy lies with how to interpret the numbers: Everyone agrees the rate of autism is rising, especially in America, but no one knows exactly why.

Those who aren't quite ready to declare an outbreak of autism say that since we now know more about the disorder, doctors are more likely to diagnose it accurately in children rather than misidentify it, and this explains why more kids seem to have it. They point to the decreasing number of children diagnosed with various forms of mental retardation—which is how many children who have unrecognized autism have been typically mislabeled—as pediatricians become more savvy at recognizing the disorder. Basically, they say children are being moved from one diagnosis to the next.

But others, who contend that this explanation can only partially account for the rise, conclude that the disorder is spreading and demand that health agencies and doctors race to find a definitive cause and a cure. What makes explaining the increase doubly difficult, according to a National Public Radio interview with Dr. Susan Folstein of the Autism Genetics Research Cooperative, is that no accurate accounting exists of what the diagnosis rates were decades ago, so it's hard to compare the numbers then and now.

However it is branded, one thing is certain: Autism isn't as rare as it was first thought to be and is, in fact, becoming one of the fastest growing developmental disorders seen in children today.

Are boys more prone to autism than girls?

Yes. Boys are four times more likely to receive a diagnosis that places them on the autistic spectrum than girls. In general, though, girls tend to exhibit a more severe form of the disorder than boys.

What are the different types of autism?

Below is a summary of four disorders commonly categorized as being on the autism spectrum. For more on how these disorders are manifested, see Chapter 3.

Classic autism: When children are diagnosed with classic autism, that means they display *significant* delays in three specific areas. First and most notable is their inability to form social relationships and/or their lack of what experts describe as a "social reciprocity," meaning they don't interact with others as typical kids do. They don't make eye contact, initiate play, or pick up on other people's cues. They may not respond when addressed—even when their name is called.

Second, they have problems communicating their thoughts and feelings to others. They may hardly use words, or use them incorrectly, or not speak at all. If they do speak, they converse in monotone, failing to infuse their sentences with emotion. They can't seem to master basic rules in conversational give-and-take, interrupting when others are talk-ing or "zoning out" in the middle of a discussion. According to a 1997 study published in the *Journal of Child Psychology and Psychiatry,* many children eventually diagnosed with autism may not have uttered a single word by the time they are two years of age. If they do, they may use the wrong words or syntax, be unable to follow complicated directions, or fail to grasp conceptual meanings behind words (they understand what a hammer is, for example, but are perplexed by the word "love").

Last, they engage in repetitive behaviors, only able to cope with day-to-day life by following strict routines, such as wearing clothes of the same color, eating only in a set pattern (as in eating a sandwich bread first, meat next, then lettuce last), or saying a phrase over and over.

All three impairments may show up at the same time, or one may be more noticeable over time. Either way, it becomes obvious to the doctor and to others who are around the child that he is hampered by all three symptoms. Children with autism are measured on a scale that ranges be-tween severe to high-functioning, depending on their development.

Asperger's Syndrome: Asperger's, as with autism in general, is far more common in boys than girls. It's actually a type of PDD, but it merits its own category because its symptoms are markedly different from those of classic autism. Because many children with Asperger's don't exhibit the complete range of obvious symptoms, it's sometimes described as a "high-functioning" form of autism. Some parents seek help much later than they ideally should because their children don't seem to be autistic to someone who is not an expert and who can of-fer a proper assessment.

Children with Asperger's do not show any deficiency in their intel-lectual abilities. In fact, some of them perform exceedingly well in school, mastering subjects and assignments as well as, if not better than, "typical" students. They also don't show any delays in language acqui-sition. They usually learn to speak at the same pace as other children, so they don't raise red flags at home and during periodic checkups at the pediatrician's office.

But there's one area in which children with Asperger's are devastat-ingly similar with other kids on the spectrum: their social life. According to the *Diagnostic and Statistical Manual of Mental Disorders,* version IV (aka *DSM–IV*), which essentially outlines in general terms the symptoms associated with mental and developmental disorders, and which is recognized as a doctor's basic diagnostic tool, Asperger's is manifested by a "qualitative impairment in social interaction" marked by at least two of the following accompanying symptoms: (a) profound lack of nonverbal behaviors such as eye contact, gestures, and facial expressions; (b) failure to develop developmentally appropriate relationships with peers; (c) a major disinterest in sharing their interests and achievements with others; and (d) deficiency in responsiveness to others. They also exhibit behaviors associated with classic autism and PDD-NOS (see below), such as hand-flapping, obsession about a specific subject matter that has caught their interest, and a pronounced need to follow set routines. They may also not be as physically coordinated as kids without autism.

What does this all mean? Asperger kids have trouble interacting with their family members, friends, teachers, and classmates. They prefer to keep to themselves, or seem unable to fit in, somehow. They may not even appear to want to try. At school, for example, they won't have one special friend to whom they're attached or want to get to know more deeply; they don't seem to know how to navigate social circles, or even care. Their faces are stoic; based on their expressions, others can't quite tell what such children are feeling. And they don't seem to have the same well of sympathy and empathy others do; if a playmate is hurt that a child with Asperger's won't share a toy, for example, that child may truly seem not to comprehend why. When asked to deviate from a schedule or a traditional way of doing something, children with Asperger's will balk because they are so committed to sticking with what they know. They also find out anything and everything there is to know about certain subjects that, for some reason, hold their interest like no other.

Pervasive Developmental Disorder Not Otherwise Specified (PDD-NOS): In a way, a diagnosis of PDD-NOS works as a catch-all for disorders that are on the autistic spectrum but don't entirely fit the labels of classic autism and Asperger's. Children who receive this diagnosis exhibit some of the behaviors associated with either classic autism or Asperger's, but miss a few significant others. For example, they possess a basic ability to gesture, which many autistic kids don't, but are unable to form intelligible sentences and remain stoic in their faces, unable to communicate their emotions, if any. Or, they are able to let their parents know when they're sad or angry, but the shifts in emotions are dramatic, showing extreme highs and lows with little gradations in between; complicated feelings such as ambivalence or nervous anticipation don't exist, only polar opposites such as overwhelming fear or reckless abandon. If they do speak, children with PDD-NOS do so with little or no emotion. They talk in the same manner whether they're happy or upset. Sentences may be stripped down to their bare essentials, without articles, prepositions, and other parts of speech.

Fragile X Syndrome: Fragile X is an inherited chromosomal abnormality that's sometimes mentioned as part of the autism spectrum. According to the advocacy group Fraxa Research Association, 20 percent of males with the disorder meet the criteria for autism. The Conquer Fragile X Foundation says 6 percent of autistic individuals have Fragile X. One in 2,000 boys is diagnosed with the syndrome, twice the number for girls. A person with Fragile X has a specific gene that isn't able to produce a protein that the brain needs to be able to learn. As a result, his mental faculties are usually severely impaired, and his moods are difficult to regulate. Children diagnosed with Fragile X typically have a long face, big ears, and flat feet, and may also suffer from epileptic seizures. Girls don't seem to suffer the same degree of mental impairment as boys, coping with a few learning disabilities instead. Unlike other forms of autism, Fragile X Syndrome can be confirmed through genetic testing.

What is Rett Syndrome and is it a type of autism?

Rett Syndrome, discovered by Austrian doctor Andreas Rett (hence the name), is a rare but serious, often fatal developmental disorder that primarily afflicts girls. Because it shares some traits with autism, the two are sometimes confused. But there are enough differences between the disorders that some experts say it is on the autism spectrum, while others stop short of labeling it as such. In the beginning, most children with Rett seem to be following the normal course of development: They learn to crawl, make tentative attempts at speaking, and appear to be just like every other toddler. At around eighteen months of age, however, these children seem to regress. They develop apraxia, a condition in which they lose control over voluntary movements such as walking or maintaining eye contact, lose skills they may have mastered, or fail to develop new ones they would've begun to explore. Although children with Rett Syndrome face enormous challenges, their prognosis isn't as bleak as it once was. Various therapies have been shown to make a difference, improving quality of life. And medications such as dopamine and opiate antagonists appear to be effective in mitigating physical symptoms. Still, there's a long way to go to finding a definitive cure for the condition.

How are children diagnosed?

Behavior specialists, therapists, and doctors assess children for autism by observation and through interviews with the children and their parents. There are a number of scales experts can use, including:

- Prelinguistic Autism Diagnostic Observation Schedule: for kids who don't talk
- Childhood Autism Rating Scale: a 15-item scale devised by staffers at

North Carolina's Treatment and Education of Autistic and related Communication handicapped CHildren (TEACCH) model, a popular intervention program
- Autism Behavior Checklist
- Checklist for Autism in Toddlers: also known as CHAT and designed for children as young as eighteen months
- Bernard Rimland's Diagnostic Checklist for Behavior-Disturbed Children: developed by the noted autism expert
- Autism Screening Instrument for Educational Planning
- Pervasive Developmental Disorder Screening Test
- Gilliam Autism Rating Scale

Most, if not all, of these scales and the many others available are based on the criteria outlined in the *DSM-IV*, which looks for the following:

- Autism: Six or more items from each of the following categories (1, 2, and 3), two of which have to come from 1, and at least one each from 2 and 3. Apart from these three categories, doctors also take into account if symptoms are present before three years of age, and if no other diagnosis better encapsulates the condition. In addition, speech therapists also employ specific tests that check for language problems associated with autism.
  1. Significant (termed "qualitative") impairment in social interaction, manifested by:
     a. Problems with eye contact, postures, facial expression, and gestures
     b. Inability to form social relationships that are appropriate to a certain age level
     c. No initiative in sharing interests, hobbies, and activities with others
     d. Unresponsiveness to another person's attempts to establish a connection
  2. Problems with communication
     a. Significant delays, or a complete inability to engage, in language development

    b. If a child speaks, a difficulty in maintaining back-and-forth communication

    c. Lack of imaginative play

  3. Repetitive and "stereotyped" patterns of behavior

    a. Obsessive and limited interest in a few subjects, sometimes to an extreme degree

    b. A strict dependence on routine, even for events that don't need it (and an inability to adjust if schedules are varied to any degree)

    c. Repetitive body movements and actions

    d. Fixation with parts of objects (and perhaps not the whole)

- Asperger's Syndrome: Experts typically look for the aforementioned symptoms, with a few exceptions. There may be little or no delay in communication skills or in cognitive development.

- PDD-NOS: Experts usually provide this diagnosis when children appear to have many of the symptoms associated with autism and Asperger's, but don't quite fit either category to a T. For example, problems may have arisen considerably later than the age of three, or problems may barely meet the criteria but cannot be explained by any other diagnosis.

What are some behaviors that could indicate that my child is autistic?

Every autistic child is different, but some of the early symptoms that parents with kids on the spectrum report include any or all of the following:

- Lack of communication, either verbally or through gestures (e.g., a child is unusually quiet or has few words in his repertoire, doesn't point or motion toward objects he likes, or won't smile or coo when someone else tries to engage him);

- Persistent hand-flapping;

- Obsessive interest in a subject or object, almost to the exclusion of others (e.g., a baby may stare at a lamp and can't be distracted from it no matter where he is in the room, or an older child may spend hours turning it on or off);
- Intense sensitivity to touch, sound, smells, or taste (e.g., a child may act as if he's being poked with nails when he comes in contact with tags from his shirt);
- Aggressive reactions, such as throwing a tantrum or banging his head, when his schedule or routine is altered in any way.

When do symptoms start to surface?

Most parents start to notice symptoms of autism at approximately two years of age or a little earlier, around the same time children are expected to be mastering language. Because language is one of the basic measures of child development, experts have a general sense of how many words kids should be able to use by age two and how much they can understand. When a two-year-old child hasn't yet spoken an intelligible word, or still speaks like a baby, parents are usually concerned enough to consult their child's pediatrician or to bring it up at a yearly checkup.

Still, some parents say they knew even earlier on that something was different about their child. You may have noticed, for example, that your little one would flinch anytime you held him in your arms, as if your touch brought him distress. Your friends may have praised your mellow baby, who would sit quietly in his bassinet or bouncy chair while you took a shower or cleaned the house, hardly uttering a peep or crying. When you pointed something out to him, he may not have followed your gaze, or may have hardly responded when you presented a spoon in front of his face as a way to entice him to eat. In truth, many parents say they had a hunch all along, and by the time the diagnosis was finally made, it was painful, but not surprising news.

What is a savant?

A savant is a person who possesses enormous intellectual abilities or talents even as they try to manage a developmental disorder. It isn't a type of autism, although autistic individuals represented in movies and on television have been depicted as savants; Dustin Hoffman's character in *Rain Man,* who was endowed with a lightning-speed ability to compute numbers, is one popular example. Savants are not just brilliant at math; they have also excelled in music and the arts, able to dig into a difficult piece of music with hardly any training, or to paint like a master. They also have impeccable recall, which they seem to access with little effort. But even among savants, there is a wide range of abilities. Some may have an impressive skill but not a rare one; for example, they may be able to draw maps well, but there are also numerous cartographers who can achieve the same degree of success in their field. Others, known as prodigious savants, have such awe-inspiring power that their gifts stand out even when compared to typically smart children and adults. Prodigious savants are extremely rare; they are the Einsteins and Michelangelos of the world who leave their mark on society for years to come.

Are all autistic children geniuses?

No. When autistic kids are called geniuses, savant syndrome has been mistaken for autism. Although the two disorders are often associated with each other, only 10 percent of people who are autistic are also diagnosed with savant syndrome. The term "genius" doesn't connote autism, either. Many geniuses display no developmental disorders whatsoever, and are merely blessed with heightened intellectual prowess.

Do all autistic children share the same traits?

Yes and no. Because there are specific symptoms and behaviors doctors search for when assessing children for autism, they do display similar traits. They all encounter difficulties when interacting with others; many hardly speak; they find learning how to communicate a challenge; most have trouble bonding with parents, caregivers, and friends. Many kids prefer to do things strictly by routine; they gravitate to the activities, objects, and topics they like and will persist in participating in them, shunning anything that falls outside their realm of interest.

Autism is a spectrum disorder, meaning that individuals who have it manifest the disorder in many varied ways. They also don't all suffer from mental retardation, for example; some are considered high-functioning and excel in academic work, while others may find even simple educational programs hard to comprehend or master. Some may suffer from an intense dislike of being touched or hearing loud noises or sitting in a crowded room (all examples of sensory issues) while others have no problems of that kind at all. One group of children may exhibit a fanatical interest over one or two beloved subjects (say, train travel or weather patterns) while another group may not be quite as obsessive.

Experts who study autism say that up to twenty genes may play a part in determining how a person will develop autism and in what way it will surface. In one child, a certain set of genes may be the culprit; in another, an entirely different group could be at play. Soon, researchers hope to be able to get more definitive answers. The Autism Genetic Resource Exchange, a project sponsored by the Cure Autism Now Foundation, is trying to unscramble the combinations to find out how family history influences the course of the developmental disorder.

Even if one compares two kids who have received remarkably similar diagnoses of a moderate-to-severe autism, they will appear just as different as they are alike. They can't be grouped into one lump, and shouldn't be. One of the hallmarks of a solid, reputable intervention program is how individual it was designed to be; because each child is different, a one-size-fits-all approach works poorly and isn't sustained in the long term.

Unfortunately, though, many people find it easy to assume that children with disabilities are all the same, defining them by their challenges rather than their distinct personalities, which is a disservice to the children.

Can autism be misdiagnosed?

Like many disorders, especially ones that can't be confirmed by a test (such as using blood or other methods), autism can be misdiagnosed. Doctors are learning new ways to spot the developmental disorder early on, but there aren't very many hard-and-fast rules. Diagnostic criteria change, and they're usually dependent on the interpretation of the expert performing the evaluation. What makes identification of autism particularly murky is that autism is a constellation of symptoms, some of which are disorders on their own. A pediatrician may think a child has autism when in reality he has sensory disorder issues only. A toddler may have other speech impediments that make it difficult to sound out words but is not autistic, or the child may simply be experiencing delays that he'll overcome in his own timeline.

Because many children often face a host of challenges (for example, showing little interest in communicating, being extra sensitive to light, or unable to sit still), doctors evaluating a child for autism look primarily for an inability to connect socially with others, which is the biggest hallmark for the developmental disorder. If social interaction is a minor problem, and the child's inability to experience downtime is an overwhelming concern, he may receive a different diagnosis altogether. That's why some parents feel it's necessary to get a second opinion, which is completely understandable. It's best, however, to seek the opinion of pediatricians and child psychologists who are familiar with autism and who have interacted extensively with autistic kids. Such professionals stand a better chance of diagnosing your child correctly and in a timely manner so they can provide the help needed as soon as possible.

If I have more children, will they be autistic, too?

Possibly. An experienced genetic counselor is the best person to assess your genetic history as well as your partner's, but if you already have one autistic child, compared to the general population, you may run a slightly higher risk of your next child being autistic as well. Studies looking into the patterns of autism are ongoing, but findings to date do point to a fairly strong genetic component. Research done on twins showed that identical twins who share the same genes were anywhere from 60 to 95 percent likely both to have autism. Other research has placed the number at 50 percent. Among fraternal twins and siblings, the recurrence rate (chance that the disorder will show up) is only 5 to 8 percent.

As there's no definitive cause for autism, it's difficult to be exact about such numbers. Among the many theories about what causes the disorder, not one of them can explain the occurrence rate we're seeing now.

Is there a cure for autism?

Unfortunately, as of this writing, there is no known cure. This should come as no surprise, however, considering that a cause has been difficult to pinpoint. Some so-called experts may claim they've found the antidote, and certain regimens may very well mitigate most symptoms, but experts agree on no solution and, whatever the treatment, kids don't disappear from the spectrum. Every year, scientists have made strides in their research, finding better ways to understand the disorder and, in turn, teaching parents, doctors, and educators more useful ways to help autistic children and adults. Advocacy groups continue to call for better funding from public and private institutions so that researchers can continue their work and find a definitive solution to this growing problem.

Although the proverbial "magic pill" is yet to be formulated, all is not hopeless. NFL superstar Dan Marino knows firsthand what it's like to begin the journey lost and confused, only to end up a decade later feeling blessed. His son, Mike, no longer exhibits any symptoms of autism; now a teenager, his life is filled with the concerns that plague most kids his age— trying out for sports teams, making the grade at school, doing his chores. "I won't say I have been cured because you can't really be cured of autism," Mike told *CBS SportsLine* in a 2002 interview, "but I have overcome it. That's what you can do—you can overcome it. I don't notice it at all anymore." Perhaps, someday, many other children will overcome autism completely. The struggle continues but there's reason to hope.

2.

CAUSES

. . . .

This is one of the most basic questions you'll ask about autism, and yet it's the one that has incited the most debate: What's the root of this developmental condition called autism? Answers run the gamut from heredity to environmental factors. In this chapter, we'll explain how science and medicine weigh in on the subject.

What causes autism?

No one knows for sure. Discussions of possible causes are highly charged, mainly because many theories abound, from the absurd to the probable. Scientists are hard at work trying to make sense of the disorder, and have made progress toward defining it and parsing its genetic makeup, but isolating a cause, or a number of causes, is still elusive.

And it's no surprise: Autism is a mysterious and tricky condition, unlike many other disorders that surface in childhood. It has so many variations, and each individual diagnosed with it presents in a different way, meaning that one person has a collection of symptoms and behaviors that don't usually match those found in another. There's no way to test for it (before a child is born or after), and kids are diagnosed primarily through observation.

The lack of information about what causes autism is disturbing, but with so many parents and organizations clamoring for answers, a solution may not be all that far off. Unfortunately, many self-crowned experts have come out of the woodwork claiming to have found the ultimate cause and hawking an accompanying cure. Although it's tempting to believe them, it's important to exercise caution when subscribing to various hypotheses, because that's all they are at this point—conjecture and assumptions that the autism research community hasn't entirely backed. Now more than ever, it's important to be your own best advocate: Keep an open mind but be a healthy skeptic.

Do vaccines cause autism?

While some researchers contend that vaccines are to blame for the increasing rates of autism, most experts believe otherwise. A study published in the British medical journal *The Lancet,* spearheaded by Dr. Andrew Wakefield, mentioned the measles-mumps-rubella (MMR) vaccine as a possible offender, but that conclusion has since been discredited, and many of the researchers who worked on this theory admitted to some errors in their findings. According to Dr. Neil Halsey of the Institute of Vaccine Safety at the Johns Hopkins University Bloomberg School of Public Health, who elaborated on the vaccine question at a National Public Radio *Talk of the Nation* program in 2003, there were numerous flaws in the way the *Lancet* study was done. In fact, a study later published in the *New England Journal of Medicine* went over the same data and found no absolute proof of any direct connection between the MMR vaccine and autism. Danish scientists examined approximately 400,000 children who received the MMR and, comparing them to thousands who did not, saw very little difference in the rates of autism between the two groups.

Another subgroup of the anti-vaccine lobby points to thimerosal, a preservative used in some vaccines (but interestingly enough, not in the suspect MMR), as the autism-causing agent. They say that methyl mercury, a poisonous substance found in thimerosal, may be what's affecting children. After all, the Food and Drug Administration does caution parents about exposing their kids to mercury; the agency goes so far as to recommend that pregnant women and those of childbearing age limit the amount of seafood they include in their diet; some types of fish are even prohibited because the agency has deemed them potentially harmful to a developing fetus. Plus, some doctors say that the symptoms of methyl mercury poisoning mimic that of autism; other experts disagree.

An article published in 2004 in the magazine *Mother Jones* examined the link between methyl mercury and autism, and went a step further in explaining what may be the connection. Rather than provoke a developmental chain of events simply by introducing mercury into a child's system, the mercury in vaccines may have been the proverbial "straw that broke the camel's back" for those children who already have a problem excreting the substance from their bodies. Scientists who subscribe to this theory believe that a number of kids diagnosed with autism may have had too much mercury in their blood, some of which may have been contributed by vaccines; they were unable to get rid of it like most children, and so developed autism as a result.

Given that there are no comprehensive, long-term studies that have examined the direct link between mercury and autism, it's difficult to wholeheartedly embrace this hypothesis. (Researchers are, however, hard at work as of this writing on a number of studies sponsored by reputable organizations such as the Centers for Disease Control.) That said, the theory accounts for only a small number of children who have autism (not everyone has a problem leaching mercury out of the bloodstream). Besides, thimerosal has been abandoned by most, if not all, vaccine makers, yet autism rates are still rising. Also, methyl mercury is also found in seafood; who's to say that what affected one particular child is the thimerosal-laced vaccine and not some fish or shellfish consumed during pregnancy by the mother, or other mercury-laden toxins to which she, or later her child, may have been unwittingly exposed?

Other events preceding the onset of autism could also be similarly blamed. But it's easier to focus on when a child was immunized rather than trace every meal the child may have eaten, every place she may have visited, or every toy she handled. Retracing the steps is daunting, because danger could have lurked anywhere. Then again, perhaps there was no environmental danger at all. It's all one big question mark, which makes the experience especially confusing for those who are nearest and dearest to the child with the diagnosis.

My child didn't exhibit any developmental problems until after he had an adverse reaction after being immunized. Is there a connection?

This is a highly controversial issue. Some parents claim that they can trace their child's problems to a period soon after vaccines were administered; they say that before their toddler went in for a regularly scheduled appointment with the pediatrician and received the usual spate of shots, she was a typical baby, observant and interested in the world. However, it's highly doubtful that there's a link. It's just that symptoms of autism tend to appear during the same period of time in which children receive the bulk of their shots. And adverse effects can and have been known to result from vaccinations, including irritability and fever. But it's never been proven beyond doubt that vaccines cause children to stop speaking or learning; that they suddenly bring on an inability to interact with others in a child who was previously a social creature; that they encourage obsessive behaviors that are common among autistic kids; or that they trigger autism.

Should I skip vaccines in the future?

We would advise against skipping vaccinations, unless of course you have religious reasons for doing so or simply don't believe in the practice and have discussed your opinion at length with your child's pediatrician. The value of vaccines far outweighs the value of any conjecture that they cause harm. For decades—in some cases even centuries—deadly or destructive communicable diseases such as polio and diphtheria endangered many children, and the advent of vaccines helped put a stop to their spread and saved many lives. But if everyone who heard that vaccines were dangerous began skipping them now, diseases that were virtually obliterated could regain a foothold, reviving old public health hazards. This doesn't mean, however, that you can't exercise caution.

Also, some pediatricians caution against having your child immunized when she's unwell—if she's running a fever, for example, or has the flu. If your child is sick, her immune system is already compromised, leaving your child vulnerable to adverse reactions such as irritability and low-grade fever, so it's best to reschedule your appointment for when she's well. And it goes without saying that if you suspect that your child has suffered due to a vaccination, you have recourse in programs run by government agencies such as the Vaccine Injury Compensation Program (www. hrsa.gov/osp/vicp).

Can you "catch" autism?

No. Autism isn't an illness; it's a developmental disorder. It isn't brought on by bacteria, nor is it spread from one individual to the next by a virus. Unfortunately, however, you may meet individuals who may distance themselves from your child, or want to shield their kids from yours, as if autism were catching. It's distressing when faced with such behavior, but chalk it up to ignorance. Many people don't understand what autism is about, and when they don't see any physical disabilities, they may assume that your child is simply "misbehaving" and will steer their children elsewhere. (For more on how to handle the reactions of strangers, see Chapter 6.)

My child was born prematurely. Does this have anything to do with her autism?

Premature babies, because they're born much earlier than the usual term of pregnancy and may not have developed all their systems as well as full-term infants, are prone to suffer many health concerns and delays. In fact, it's customary that when children are born weeks early, pediatricians will expect their development to lag somewhat accordingly. For example, if your child was born five weeks early, she may walk five (or more) weeks later than others her age.

During the last few months of gestation, babies grow at an amazing rate; their lungs are maturing, their hearts and brains are developing, and they're putting on fat in preparation for life outside the womb. When that entire process is truncated, development is also cut short. Premature babies are birthed with neurological problems, are unable to control their body temperature, or even take their first breath unassisted by machines.

That said, it's difficult to say whether autism is caused by prematurity. It's possible that some of their neurological challenges can be attributed to being born too soon, but many babies who reach the entire forty weeks of pregnancy develop the disorder, too. To date, no direct correlation has been established between premature birth and autism. It's possible to see, though, how it may have an effect on a child's ability to master certain skills later in life.

Can a child develop autism from severe dietary allergies?

Most medical experts who treat children with autism don't believe so. Still, there are those who claim that autism is caused by allergies; they say autistic individuals with serious sensitivities have weakened immune systems that can't process yeast, bacteria, and certain proteins in specific food products. But the studies cited to bolster this position don't actually prove an unambiguous correlation; mostly they show that a number of autistic children also suffer from food sensitivities. In some people, food allergies can be caused by their bodies' inability to metabolize certain substances. But no studies definitively establish that an allergic condition can make children autistic, and most also invite further questions. For example, if specific food allergies were to cause autism, why do many children who are on the spectrum appear to not have sensitivities to anything they eat? If food allergies are to blame, why aren't all children with severe food allergies autistic?

Many autistic children suffer from severe allergies to certain food products, but it's unlikely the disorder can be attributed to them. It's more plausible that the two conditions coexist, one exacerbating the other.

When a person develops an allergy, the body reacts to a certain substance—called an allergen—that irritates its cells, which then release antihistamine and cause inflammation. If she has an aversion to a number of ingredients—gluten, for example—and inadvertently eats something that contains it, her digestive system becomes uncomfortable; she may feel pain in her abdominal area, turn gassy, and generally feel under the weather. Now, if she's also autistic and doesn't feel well, it makes sense that some of her behaviors usually associated with the developmental disorder may become heightened; if she normally flaps her hands and is frightened by loud noises, if her allergy is bothering her she may react even *more* vehemently when confronted with sounds she doesn't like. If she likes to spin endlessly to feel more in control of her surroundings, she may do so in full force when she's feeling unwell. But this is true even in individuals without autism; when we're ill, we don't act like our usual selves. We're irritable and grow tense easily. All we want is to feel better, find comfort, and be left alone.

What is the link between folic acid and autism?

Some camps insist that autism can be traced back to a woman's intake of folic acid, a nutrient that metamorphoses—especially during pregnancy—into a B vitamin called "folate." For decades, expectant moms didn't ingest enough folic acid, and thousands of children were born with birth defects that could have been prevented. But now that this supplement is available in many fortified breads, cereals, and grain products as recommended by the Food and Drug Administration, critics claim that the problem may now be that pregnant women may have too much of it in their diet, and as a result, give birth to autistic children. Detractors of this opinion say that no one has adequately examined the negative effects of introducing such a nutrient in the American food supply, and that it may be the cause of autism's rising rates.

Although the idea is intriguing (as are many of the hypotheses about the cause of autism), no direct correlation between folic acid and autism has been established, and to date there have been no studies confirming this theory. Scientists agree that the matter bears examination, but the Food and Drug Administration isn't as concerned because the agency claims it was diligent in its research and found no reason to change its folic acid recommendations. Indeed, the nutrient has proven to be a powerful weapon in the fight to prevent neural tube defects and anencephaly in babies. In addition, some autism experts believe that prescribing higher doses of folic acid is a viable way to treat children with autism; this, however, has not been proven in controlled studies, so many experts are cautious about following this treatment route.

Is autism genetic?

Experts now believe, and research proves them right, that there's a strong genetic component to the developmental disorder. But rather than one gene being responsible for the development of autism, as in Rett Syndrome, a handful of genes may contribute to the condition. More work needs to be done in the field to clarify exactly what happens with the genes and when.

However, genetics alone clearly cannot explain why autism occurs. Bloodlines simply cannot account for every single person who has been evaluated and deemed to be autistic. In many families with more than one child, siblings do not develop the illness. Or, in charting genetic history, neither side of the family tree has had any children who were diagnosed autistic or shown symptoms that could be attributed to the disorder. That's why many researchers think that external forces are also to blame. But what those forces are specifically is still up for debate, hence the proliferation of theories about what causes autism, ranging from vaccinations to environmental toxins.

Is there anything I could have done to cause my child to develop the disorder?

No matter what happens to your child, it's important to avoid placing the blame on your own shoulders. When your child is the one suffering, it's normal for you to look to yourself as the person responsible, however unpleasant, because doing so allows you to feel some measure of control over what's essentially an uncontrollable situation. It allows you to help make sense of a disorder that elicits so many questions and so few answers.

It's also especially easy for you to tap into your guilt when ideas that purport to explain how children develop autism seemingly appear out of the blue. Many such theories appear to point to actions we made as parents—not resting enough during pregnancy and therefore possibly bringing on preterm labor, or agreeing to a doctor's suggestion that a child get vaccinated—actions that, if they could be undone, would supposedly avert the onslaught of autism. The truth is, these suggestions are not that much different from the old thinking doctors had about "refrigerator moms." The implication was that if a mother had done a better job of connecting with her baby from the outset, autism would've been avoided, as if autism were like a wayward car in oncoming traffic, something a parent could spot easily.

But we now know that mother-child bonding doesn't dictate whether a baby will someday develop autism, and current science doesn't support many theories that claim to explain the cause of autism. The condition affects children from all backgrounds, regardless of race, wealth, or education. You didn't do anything to cause it or bring it on. Instead of pointing a finger at yourself, you deserve praise for committing yourself to finding ways to help your child have a better life. You are, after all, your child's best advocate; she relies on you for support and guidance.

3.

MANIFESTATIONS

. . . .

Just like other kids, children living with autism are unique in their own way. While many exhibit similar symptoms, others will find themselves struggling with their own set of challenges. Learn what those are and how you can help them manage the difficulties.

Why won't my child look me in the eye?

Lack of eye contact is so common among autistic children that it's one of the first symptoms doctors look for when evaluating patients. There are a few different schools of thought to explain why your child won't maintain eye contact. Some experts suggest your child can't look you in the eye because he hasn't learned that this is an important way to communicate. He hasn't learned to understand facial expressions, so he doesn't try to "read" you when you speak or respond to him.

Researchers at the University of London–Birkbeck found that babies who were only two days old exhibited some basic ability to form eye contact. As they get older, nonautistic kids only get better at it, taking their cues from another person's eyes and face to be able to discern what they're thinking and feeling. But an autistic child can't do this. It may be that your child's brain is wired differently, so when he looks at you, he's not able to register what you're trying to communicate through your eyes. He may also be aware of this but can't respond appropriately by looking back at you. Instead his perception is jumbled, or worse, he may feel so deluged by input from the look in your eyes, the set of your mouth, the flash of your grin, or tilt of your head that it's too intense for him to hold your gaze. He looks away instead, or stares at something less overwhelming, such as the floor or a blank wall.

Why does my child look off to the side and avert his gaze a lot?

What you're observing is a visual problem that affects many autistic children. Your child is glancing at the periphery often because he may have trouble managing the movement of his eyes. He may be unable to look straight ahead at a person or object, so he observes it from the side or quickly glances at it, feels overwhelmed by the visual input, then looks away and repeats the same action until he's figured out what he's looking at. No wonder many autistic children have difficulty learning when so much of what we know is based on what we see. Talk to an ophthalmologist or optometrist who's familiar with the condition; these professionals may be able to outfit your child with the proper glasses to help him coordinate his eye movements.

Why can't my child read my facial expressions correctly?

You may notice that your child reacts in unexpected ways to your gestures and facial expressions. For example, if you smile, he may run away as if you had frowned at him; if he is throwing a tantrum in public and you give him a severe look to indicate your disapproval, it has no effect. The answer may lie in the brain. In a British study published in the journal of neurology, *Brain,* scientists discovered that people with autism process facial expressions differently from those without autism, even if they are similar in many significant ways such as age and IQ level. Their brain activity registers dissimilar patterns and they exhibit an abnormal structure in the cerebellum, a part of the brain located at the base of the skull that is responsible for coordinating the body's movements. This means that people with autism may not interpret faces the same way as those who aren't autistic. Doctors also saw abnormal activity in the medial temporal lobe, which, among many other tasks, receives input from the senses, manages responses to them, and serves as the center for memory. Moreover, other parts of the brain that process facial expressions aren't as active in those with autism compared to participants not so diagnosed.

Another reason your child may not be interpreting your expressions correctly may be that he or she is likely focusing on other parts of your face that send confusing information about what you may be trying to say. A study in progress at Yale University is finding that autistic kids tend to look at the mouth more than the eyes. Unfortunately, the mouth isn't as accurate or precise a communicator of thoughts and emotions as the eyes. Kids also can't seem to recognize separate parts of the face and attribute them to one specific person; only when the parts are combined to make one recognizable whole can autistic kids more easily distinguish one face from the next.

It may help you relate with how your child is feeling if you try this exercise: Think back to your last job interview. You likely tried to maintain eye contact, knowing it's expected of you, but found it uncomfortable or overwhelming for any number of reasons, including your discomfort with the interviewer, or your general nervousness about applying for a job. You see him frowning and fear he's not impressed by your résumé. You see him purse his lips as you answer and you interpret this as a signal that he's underwhelmed by your talent. So instead of looking at your potential boss's face, you glance around the room, whether or not you're aware that you're doing so to minimize your discomfort. In a way, that's what your autistic child may be doing by not looking at you; he may be attempting to cope with overwhelming input and anxiety, and this is the only way he knows how.

Why won't our child speak?

Simply put, your child isn't talking because he can't. That doesn't mean his vocal cords are faulty, although he may have problems that will require the help of a speech therapist. It also doesn't mean he can't comprehend you. It just means that he's unable to let you know what he's thinking, feeling, or experiencing through words. Some parents who first learn about the diagnosis think their child doesn't speak simply because he doesn't want to, but that's not the case with an autistic child. Communication isn't merely a task he is avoiding because he wants to be difficult. That said, many parents report success of varying degrees in getting their kids to talk once the youngsters are enrolled in a consistent and reputable intervention program. Some early childhood development programs geared toward autistic children begin to teach them how to communicate through gestures and sign language, then move on toward speech.

Why does my child not play with his toys properly?

One of the symptoms of the disorder that parents notice first is that their child doesn't play with toys "correctly," or the way he's expected to. For instance, your child may line up puzzle pieces instead of putting them together. In fact, all he may do with his toys—cars, balls, stuffed animals—is line them up, regardless of their function. Or, he'll play with them in a manner that you've never seen before, like occupying himself for long stretches of time twisting and handling the string of a yo-yo instead of tossing it up and down as is customary. Some kids may even disregard toys altogether. Lining up toys is a form of *stimming,* a visual technique that may make him feel more assured that his world is in perfect order. Or it may comfort him better to see that his toys are arranged just so. Also, if your child (like many other autistic kids) is unable to participate in imaginative play, a developmental skill necessary to fully enjoy many toys, he might be having difficulty grasping complicated concepts. Take the aforementioned puzzle—how can your child complete a puzzle (let alone start it) if he can't even conceptualize that what he's assembling is supposed to look like the picture on the box? Or that the seemingly random pieces do indeed fit together? To him, it may all be a jumble, so stacking them up or arranging them in rows is a simple way to use them.

Autistic children are challenged by representational play. If in an attempt to engage him in pretend play, you roar at your child like a bear, he may think you're trying to hurt him and run away. In fact, autism expert and scientist Simon Baron-Cohen, in a study he led in 1992, concluded that if babies and toddlers don't appear able to participate in symbolic play, they're likely to be diagnosed with autism later in life.

What is echolalia?

When your child repeats apparently meaningless words and phrases uttered by somebody else, he's exhibiting echolalia, as in "to echo." He may duplicate something he heard the day before or perhaps weeks, months, even years earlier. He may even follow a certain pattern of speech, or replay a snippet of dialogue over and over, down to the intonation or accent. Echolalia isn't limited to a few words; your child may be able to recite a song's lyrics completely, or sing it in the same way a musician has recorded it. He may also be able to relay an entire conversation, including pauses and changes in volume, without understanding completely what the exchange meant.

Many children with ASD (autism spectrum disorder) use echolalia without intending to communicate. For example, your child may repeat words that absolutely have no context given what's happening at the present time (you ask him if he wants juice, and he says "Don't walk on the grass," for example), or he may sound like he's talking to himself, as Dustin Hoffman's character, Ray, did in the movie *Rain Man,* when he would say, "Gotta watch Wapner" out of the blue.

But echolalia could also signal that your child is taking baby steps on the road to communication. In fact, echolalia is normal in some cases; babies, for example, routinely engage in echolalia (a parent says "mama," and the baby repeats it, not knowing it means his mother). It's an infant's way of grasping the complicated nuance and ritual of language, and as kids who aren't on the spectrum begin to master communication, echolalia dissipates and is replaced by more direct responses—the back-and-forth of language takes over. On the other hand, a child with autism becomes stalled in the echolalia stage. With luck, the stasis lasts only for a while, but without early or intensive intervention, it may persist much longer.

You can tell if your child is trying to communicate with echolalia if what he's saying seems to be in response to you or to the situation before him. Enamored of the movie *Dinosaur,* four-year-old Alex Ham-Kucharski took a liking to the line, "Stand together," which was a verbal signal for a herd to assemble. When Alex went to the mall or went trick-

or-treating and saw a group of people, he'd yell out, imitating the dinosaur's voice, "Stand together." At first, it was disconcerting for his parents, until they realized he was merely trying to recognize a group, connecting it to what he had previously seen in the movie, in an effort to urge them to converge in the way he'd witnessed onscreen. It was a clunky way to let people know what he was thinking, but it was actually a positive sign that a previously nonverbal autistic child was branching out. Years later, Alex grew out of echolalia and was able to communicate his thoughts more clearly. If he wanted people to line up, he'd simply say, "Line up," without using the intonation of a growling, animated dinosaur.

What does it mean when a child "stims"?

Many autistic children stim, which means they engage in repetitive, self-stimulatory behaviors, either by moving objects or their bodies in a certain way. For example, a child may bounce a ball repeatedly against the wall or pick at his cuticles incessantly. He may tap a specific beat over and over or spin until he's dizzy. Hand-flapping is so common among autistic kids that it's almost synonymous with the disorder. Doctors have varying explanations for stimming. Some say it's a way for a child to gain control over his environment; if he finds a place too loud, crowded, or enclosing, to feel calmer he may engage in his favorite stimming behavior.

It may be upsetting to you to see your child stim; you may think it makes him look troubled or draws attention to his autism. Instead, think of it as his signal, whether he's aware he's sending it or not, that he may not be feeling entirely comfortable with his surroundings; he may also do it more often when he's exhausted. This is helpful to you because you can then take his cue and try to figure out what may be upsetting him, and help him work through it. You may be able to remove the unsettling object or condition, or lead your child to a place that feels safer to him.

If the environment seems to be the way he likes it, there may be other reasons for his stimming. He could be hyposensitive, a sensory dysfunction that indicates his sense of touch isn't as attuned as others. Somehow, the brain in a hyposensitive child has trouble processing the tactile input—or whatever it is that's touching him—so in order for him to "feel" the object, he has to rub it or touch it more often or more strongly than would children without autism.

It's important to know that autistic children do not all share the same stimming behaviors. If your child likes to rock back and forth, his friend who's also on the spectrum may not. It's also not necessarily a measure by which you can compare whether your child's autism is milder or more severe than someone else's.

In a way, many of us who aren't autistic may indulge in stimming behaviors from time to time. If you're stuck in traffic and are growing aggravated by the minute, you may find yourself twirling your hair because it feels relaxing. This is similar to what your child does if, for example, he rubs his fingers together anytime he has to ride a crowded bus. The difference between you and your child is that you may not necessarily twirl your hair every single time you need to relax—you wouldn't do it at a high-powered meeting at the office, for example, because you're aware that you have to appear professional and composed, and you've learned other ways to cope with tension. Or, you'd simply tell a colleague you're nervous about your upcoming presentation and reduce your anxiety verbally.

For many reasons, a child with autism can't easily communicate what he's feeling. He may not even know exactly what he's feeling in the first place. So for him, it's not simple to substitute one behavior for the next. With guidance from a knowledgeable therapist, sensory integration expert, or your child's autism-savvy doctor, you'll be able to help him come up with more appropriate ways to find comfort in his world. Instead of screeching loudly and flapping his hands at a scary noise, he may learn to cover his ears. Rather than hit a playmate because she's coming too close to him, he'll learn, with your help and patience, that he can walk to a corner, and rub his own arm gently to calm himself down. Or he may even let go of his stimming behavior entirely, once he's able to communicate better with the world.

What does it mean when a child "perseverates"?

To perseverate means to repeat. An autistic child may uncontrollably repeat a word, phrase, or gesture even after the stimulus that triggered the response has stopped. The behavior is similar to stimming, in the sense that your child engages in repetitive movements, and many kids with "classic autism" perseverate.

Perseveration also refers to an obsession or fixation about an idea, method, interest, person, or object. For example, your child may insist on doing something in the same way: His toy cars must be "parked" around his room based on his own specifications; he eats his lunch in a specific pattern (juice first, then fries, followed by a perfectly round cookie); he may only be able to watch TV shows that have to do with vehicles or dinosaurs and nothing else, and if you stray from that, he may respond in a manner you don't quite understand or know how to manage, like kicking the screen or rolling on the floor until you find a show that features the subjects on which he's perseverating. Like many other children, he may only want to read the same book, or eat the same foods, except in his case it's much harder, maybe even nearly impossible, to coax him to try something new.

What are "comfort zones"?

We all have comfort zones, which are generally defined by the areas in life or in the activities we engage in that make us feel at ease. If you're not autistic, your comfort zone may cut a wide swath: You feel relaxed if you live in a neighborhood in a small town where the residents are friendly and the houses aren't set too close together, prefer a nine-to-five job where you can predict your daily schedule fairly accurately, and have a home that is spacious, neat, and clean. As long as those parameters are met, you're fine. But if you're plucked out of this setting and are taken, say, to New York City where you live in a cramped, boxy apartment dating back to the 1920s (and looks it, too) and are forced to work freelance with a schedule that shifts every day, you'd feel stressed and completely out of your element. Given time, you may get used to the new rhythms of your life, and may even welcome the changes.

Your autistic child has comfort zones, too, but they may be much narrower. He may have specific wants and needs that have to be met for him to feel happy. He may not just prefer an airy room but an empty one, at that. He may not just need lots of light but a certain kind of light (incandescent versus fluorescent, for example). Instead of feeling comfortable when he's around small groups, he may also require that the group comprise only people he's familiar with. The definition of his comfort zone may be highly detailed, and the rules may not necessarily be that easy for you to discern.

Just like you, your autistic child needs to have his comfort zones respected, even if they don't make sense to others. You may not understand why a simple pat on the back would send him into hysteria, but if for him a complete lack of physical contact feels best, try to respect his wishes. Comfort zones expand and change over time, and as your child receives help from therapists and other autism experts, his will widen too, and he will become able to accommodate a bigger and more complex world. And when that happens, he'll be able to grasp new skills, which will help further widen his zone, and each will build on the other.

What is sensory integration dysfunction?

We learn about the world through the information we receive from our five senses, which our brain and central nervous system put together and interpret to give us a coherent whole. Say, for example, we enter a restaurant to have dinner. We see the long line in front of the reservation desk and the people milling about, looking forlorn and impatient; we hear the noise of a roomful of diners; we smell the food cooking and trays of meals hoisted by the bustling wait staff; our mouths water in anticipation, and because all the seats are taken we lean against the wall and feel it uncomfortable against our backs as we wait. The result? Some of us decide the restaurant is obviously too busy and so we leave; others may patiently remain, having decided that a busy place like that probably serves good food so it's worth the hassle. Either way, we are able to take in everything around us and use the input to make decisions about our actions.

When a child has sensory integration issues, as many autistic kids do, they have difficulty processing information they receive from their senses. Their minds are unable to integrate all the sensations and interpret them, creating confusion. They may also have difficulty with individual senses— some are overdeveloped, heightening every input received from that source of information, and others may be underdeveloped, muting that source. It's hard to know what your child is experiencing, but suffice it to say his sensory pathways aren't giving him all the data he needs to be able to behave as others. His brain, which in a sense acts as a gatekeeper, allowing some input to get through and others to be filtered out, also may not be able to rank the stimuli he's receiving, meaning he can't discriminate between what's relevant and irrelevant, and focus on what's important.

Your child, for example, may enter the same room described above and have the following experience: The long line that meets him upon entering the door doesn't appear like a handful of strangers. Instead, it may look like an army closing in on him because that's how his brain is processing what he sees. The colors of other people's clothing may be so garishly bright they hurt his eyes, or may be so pale that they blend together and he can't differentiate one from the other. The din from the restaurant may, to his ears, sound as raucous as a rock concert even though everyone's speaking in conversational tones. Or the noise may seem so eerily low to him that he grows uncomfortable because it sounds as if everyone around him is whispering and, try as he might, he just doesn't understand. The extra saliva produced in his mouth from hunger may feel so uncomfortable to him that he wants to spit. And the wall on which he may lean on feels so heavy against his back that he seems to be glued to it and he won't be able to get away. Or he may hardly feel the floor at all because his mind can't register the feel of the carpet, and he feels as if he's sinking into a vacuum, and all he can do to stay level is stomp.

If it isn't his surroundings that are bothering him, it may be the label on his shirt, which feels so scratchy it's as if a sharp fork is repeatedly scraping against his skin every time he moves. And even if no one sense is overpowering him, taken as a whole they may be bombarding him with so much information that everything is jammed together into one overwhelming chunk. He can't settle into the wait, for instance, if he's registering everything all at once: the clang of silverware against plates, the feel of the carpet underfoot, the crowd gathering at the front, the sensations of his tongue in his mouth, the smell of cooking wafting from the kitchen. It may feel like an unsettling sensory assault.

Given all this, how can he sit still patiently in such a chaotic (or so it seems to him) environment? How can he focus on the yummy dinner he's about to sit down for when his feet feel like they're walking on quicksand? How can he respond in the same way you would? That explains why your child may seem like he's acting up—his senses aren't functioning like yours.

What are tactile, vestibular, and proprioceptive dysfunctions?

Children with autism often have sensory integration dysfunction in three different systems:

- *Tactile:* Our skin is lined with nerve endings that send messages to the brain so we know what it is we're touching. That's how we know when we're feeling hot, cold, pain, pleasure, and pressure. In turn, we know how to respond to touch; we know to pull away if we get near a hot stove, for example, or to wear a coat when it's cold outside. But if your child has sensory integration issues, his sense of touch is impaired. He may flinch if you pat his back softly, perceiving it as a hard blow. Or he may insist on walking barefoot on the summer-scorched pavement because he doesn't quite register the searing heat.
- *Proprioceptive:* This system controls the movements of the body and allows us to know how body parts are positioned in relation to one another. It allows you to move naturally and fluidly; your body senses

where you are and shifts accordingly. An autistic person who has a dysfunction in this area may have sensory receptors that can't read these signals, and so his movements seem jerky or uncoordinated. Or he may not know to keep his distance from other people (hence his continual violation of personal space) because he doesn't have a clear perception of where his body ends and someone else's begins.

- *Vestibular:* We gain a sense of balance through the inner ear, on which this system relies, and which also takes into account gravity and the body's movements. When this system is compromised, your child's ability to sense balance and how he takes up space in the world is lost. The simple act of walking down a flight of stairs may feel dangerous, the descent too vertiginous, his equilibrium completely off. He feels unsteady at every step. If this system is underdeveloped, he may not be well attuned to changes in stability. He may twirl around incessantly because he never quite feels dizzy, or he may require that much stimulation to experience a world in balance.

Why does my child respond aggressively to others?

Aggression is one of the most difficult manifestations of autism to manage. You may be feeling overwhelmed by your child's aggression, and don't know how to face any more attacks, the most common of which are hitting, biting, and kicking. You're not alone: Not many parents can handle it, especially if the aggression is directed at you, but it may be helpful to understand where it's coming from.

Imagine that your emotions are a jumble. Feelings engulf you and you have no way to make sense of them or to let others know clearly what you want and need. When you try to communicate in the limited ways you know how, you may not get the desired results because you've been misinterpreted. And that's not all: Your physical world is an indecipherable puzzle, too. Light bothers you, and sounds seem to boom in your ear. A walk in the street isn't tranquil, as you're bombarded left and right by what you see, hear, and touch. Worse, people seem to be laughing at you, or seem offended at the things you say or do, and you don't know why. This may be your child's reality. No wonder he lashes out sometimes, perhaps out of frustration or fear, or maybe because he doesn't know any other way to react. Behavioral therapy works wonders in alleviating aggression. Talk to your child's developmental pediatrician and therapists to learn how best to handle these episodes. In extreme cases, medication may be warranted.

Why does my child hit himself?

Many autistic children engage in self-injurious behavior, which includes hitting, biting, or scratching themselves. Your child may be affected by something he hears or sees in his environment and he reacts to it by hitting himself. Or, he may simply be trying to "feel" himself or his surroundings to compensate for a sense of touch that's underdeveloped. He may be stimming and unaware of the pain, or unable to voice his emotions and exhibiting anger or frustration in this manner. Experts have come up with other reasons as well. According to Stephen Edelson, Ph.D., of the Center for the Study of Autism in Salem, Oregon, an autistic child may also derive delight from his behavior because beta-endorphins, chemicals that elicit pleasurable sensations, are released by the brain. He may also hit himself as a way to catch your attention.

Do autistic children have bigger heads?

It's true. Experts have long believed that some children with autism, specifically males, may have bigger heads than others without the disorder. These findings can't be explained by conditions marked by big heads such as hydrocephalus. The temporal lobes of autistic children may measure larger than those in typical kids. A number of these children had normal-sized heads throughout early childhood, but as they grew older, they began to develop larger-than-average heads.

Why does my child walk on his toes?

Many young children walk on their toes, but they usually outgrow it. When they don't, doctors usually watch them closely for signs of a neurological impairment such as autism. Many autistic kids have problems with their proprioceptive sensory system, the part of the brain that controls body movements, which may explain why their feet can't or don't fall into the familiar heel-to-toe motion. His vestibular system (see page 39) may be faulty, too, which may cause him to feel off-kilter unless he walks on his toes. Or, he may have an actual physical foot problem that needs to be evaluated by an orthopedist. If you'd like to know how to address toe-walking, consult a pediatrician who has experience treating children with autism and who can suggest a few exercises or interventions. If he's unable to help your child, he should recommend someone who can.

My child speaks, but why doesn't he realize that what he says is sometimes hurtful or awkward?

Nuance is a difficult concept for your child to grasp. Communication is difficult enough for those who aren't autistic, let alone for those with the disorder. (Remember the last time you inadvertently put your foot in your mouth?) Many children, regardless of whether or not they have the developmental disorder, have trouble with tact. Although your child may communicate adequately on a literal level—saying "I want to eat" when he's hungry, for example, or "let's play" when he wants to have fun—he may not grasp, let alone know how to navigate, the intricacies of social interaction. He's unable to read between the lines, or to comprehend how the person he's speaking to perceives what he's saying. To do so requires a tremendous amount of empathy, which many autistic children lack.

Emotions are slippery, and even people without autism make mistakes in interpreting what another person may be feeling. But to someone who's autistic, it's downright tough. That accounts for why your child may blurt out something in public that you would ordinarily suppress (for example, loudly exclaiming, "That lady's face is full of bumps" when he sees someone with pimples, or saying, "The soup is yucky" when you're at someone else's house for dinner). Rather than be upset by his inability to monitor what he's saying, try to take heart in his ability to say anything at all, no matter how candid or inappropriate. Many kids with ASD can't communicate verbally with others, or do so only through repetitive speech. Your child is progressing and will, with help, learn how to assess the situation and use judgment over what he says.

4.

MANAGING
YOUR EMOTIONS

. . . .

There's so much more to autism than learning how to handle the day-to-day challenges. It throws you a curve ball that can wreak havoc on your and your family's long-term emotional health. But with guidance and support, you can weather the ups and downs with confidence.

Will our lives ever be the same?

Let's be honest: You've been handed an enormous challenge. For months you nurtured a pregnancy or awaited the arrival of a lovely adopted child, and dreamed of a different kind of family life in your head. You probably envisioned dealing with the usual crises: managing the first few bumbling months of parenthood when you're still trying to figure out how to be a mom or dad; nursing your child through the first tooth, the first step, the first day at school; juggling finances so you can afford the expenses of family life; hashing out discipline issues; teaching your child how to eat healthfully, display good manners, navigate life.

Then came the diagnosis of autism, and you're suddenly plunged into a strange jungle filled with jargon—PDD, sensory integration, IEP, proprioceptive, ABA—that you have to not only sort out but *understand* so you can cope from one day to the next. Your days, at least during the early years, are filled with endless appointments with therapists, doctors, teachers, and experts. Exhausted, you spend your nights filled with a mixture of dread and hope, each emotion cycling through you like too much work. And then of course, there's also your wonderful child, so intact on the outside, but, inside, you imagine she's fractured and confused.

It's hard to say that your life will be "the same" as other families that don't have children with autism. In fact, it won't. But the alternative isn't necessarily horrible, either. It's just different. Your future can be as bright and wonderful as that of other families. The biggest challenge is to get your child the help she needs, and fast. The earlier she's placed in a program or starts a regimen that addresses her various needs—be they physical, social, or educational—the better her prognosis will be. You'll be able to build a support system, and establish a goal to ensure that your child—and in turn, the rest of your family—will be able to fashion a rewarding and wonderful life.

Your travails won't be easy. But solutions do exist for most, if not all, the problems attendant with autism. Rest assured that if you receive the proper guidance, life may not be the same, but it will be what you make it out to be. Go ahead and have a good one.

We're despondent over our child's diagnosis. What should we do?

First, allow yourself the time to mourn for the child you expected to have. There's nothing wrong or disloyal in acknowledging your grief, which is, in fact, a natural and necessary emotion. For a few weeks or months, expect to vacillate between sadness and hope, disappointment and perseverance. Ambivalence is completely appropriate at this time. Sometimes, the feelings you experience will be so intense they leave you reeling, but resist the urge to label yourself "nuts." Rather than chastise yourself for feeling terrible about the diagnosis, give yourself permission to grieve. The truth is that you have just received horrible news, but—and you must remind yourself of this—it's not a death sentence. Everybody feels the way you do, especially in the beginning.

It's important to have an outlet for your emotions, too, as bottling them up inside will only cause you to feel alone and isolated, making the experience that much more painful. Talk to your child's pediatrician; he or she may be able to put your child's future into perspective and guide you through the process of getting help. Or talk to supportive family members and friends who can lend a nonjudgmental ear or provide a warm hug when you need one. Visit the Web sites of organizations for parents of autistic children and make use of the many bulletin boards; you may find comfort in the company of other parents like yourself who are struggling to make sense of the diagnosis. Online bulletin boards are especially helpful in that they provide you the cloak of anonymity; sometimes it's easier to share your true feelings with complete strangers whom you may not see face to face. If a friendly voice is what you need, call a helpline and unburden yourself by phone. (For more information, see the Resources section at the end of this book.)

If, however, you find yourself so disheartened about the diagnosis that you're unable to break through the sadness and experience any joy, or if your emotions prevent you from performing even the most basic functions of daily life such as eating, sleeping, and caring for your child, or if you've had thoughts of suicide (even fleetingly), consult a licensed therapist or psychologist immediately. If you have any of these symptoms, you may be suffering from depression, a condition that needs professional attention. Depression isn't a sign of weakness; on the contrary, seeking the appropriate help is a testament to your personal strength and your commitment as a parent. After all, if you're not well then you won't be able to get your child the help she needs to fashion a fruitful and happy life.

How can I help my relatives process the diagnosis?

First, you need to be sure you've processed the information yourself before you'll be able to help others comprehend the enormity of the situation. By this, we don't mean you shouldn't discuss the diagnosis right away, especially if you rely on family members for guidance. Their support will be helpful, especially in the first few weeks when emotions are raw. Their encouragement will most definitely make a difference in your future, and your child's future, too.

The best weapon for tackling confusion is solid, hard facts. Take any handouts about autism your pediatrician may have provided you and distribute them among your relatives. Like you, they may harbor some misconceptions about the developmental disorder that can be clarified with basic information. Share these materials and any other books on autism so they can do some advance reading. Information is power, and you may find that simply providing them with the latest research will bring them up to date. If you're open to it, you may also want to invite one or two of your closest family members to your child's next assessment; this way, they can meet your child's doctor or therapist and ask any questions they have. (Check with your healthcare provider before bringing a guest to your next appointment, though.)

Be prepared for what may come across as insensitive or hurtful questions. Sometimes those closest to you are the ones who seem completely unaware of the pain caused by the statements that they make. In trying to make sense of a difficult situation, they may forget to pay attention to their tone or word usage. Also, expect to be bombarded with their own autism "expertise." As you may well know, the disorder has been in the news lately, and some of your relatives may feel compelled to impart what they've seen, read, or heard. It's their way of exerting control over a situation that they actually can't steer. If they offer unsolicited solutions or sound as if they're being either bossy or pushy, in all likelihood they may simply be making an effort to manage their own concerns and confusion.

Be clear about what you think will be helpful. When you break the news to them, you may be able to head off trouble at the pass by stating that you'd like for them to just listen to you and that any suggestions about treatment, cause, or intervention are best left to your child's doctors and teachers (unless, of course, your relatives have had firsthand experience of autism, in which case it's beneficial to commiserate). You may want to remind them that autism research is an ever-changing field, that new questions and answers arise every day, and only the experts can really know for sure what's been proven and what's junk science.

If your family members seem angry or sad about the news, allow them time to take in the diagnosis. Just like you, they may have held visions of what the future was to be like for your child, and now they have to reconfigure those dreams. Your parents, siblings, and in-laws may appear more affected than distant cousins, aunts, and uncles because they're close to you and feel your pain. However, your close relatives may feel awkward about letting you know that they feel your disappointment, or may not have the verbal skills to put their emotions into words eloquently. So they try, sometimes failing miserably at empathy or sympathy.

In most cases, unless you already have deep-seated conflicts with your relatives that have nothing to do with your child's autism, families do rise to the occasion. Keep the lines of communication open and, in time, you'll likely find that they'll be allies in your search for answers to your child's autism.

I've accepted that my child is autistic but my partner hasn't. What should we do?

This is a tough one. You have both experienced quite a shock, and it will take time for the news to sink in. You may have been able to rise to the occasion much more quickly than your spouse. Perhaps you were better prepared for the diagnosis because you noticed differences in your child sooner, or were more inclined to look at them without proposing alternative explanations, whereas your partner may have been more inclined to overlook them in the hope that your child would grow out of what was thought to be a "phase." Neither of you is to blame for the ways in which you try to manage adversity.

If the diagnosis is recent, give your partner time to recover. Let him or her know that you're there every step of the way. Offer assistance if your partner is befuddled by any of the information, and then step back and allow the space needed to digest it all. Sometimes our loved ones need room to grow. Remember, your partner loves your child as much as you do, even though he or she may appear ill at ease with him.

But if months have passed and your partner still seems in denial and is unwilling to help or participate in decision-making and the day-to-day management of your child's hectic schedule, it may be time to seek some professional help. You will need to be able to lean on your partner in the years ahead as you help your child find the best interventions, enroll in an appropriate school, make friends, and acquire new skills. Your child will need to know that both parents are her champions, no matter where she stands on the autistic spectrum. Friends, relatives, and even strangers will need to see that your family is a united front, at peace with the diagnosis and ready to take on challenges, so they can take their cues from you. Your partner will need to have that same peace within him- or herself, too, in order to figure out how to forge a strong relationship with your child.

A couples therapist, a counselor, or a religious advisor may help you communicate with each other about your fears and concerns for the future. Sharing such concerns in a safe place where each of you is respected and accepted by a neutral third party, one who has experience helping families like yours, can help both of you accept that your child is autistic. A counselor may also help you make sense of any resentment you feel about your partner's inability to adapt as quickly as you have; you'll be able to express your emotions in a positive way so healing can begin.

Also, give your partner room to take the lead in some aspect of your child's medical and therapeutic regimens. You may find it difficult to let go of the reins, especially if your partner's been hands-off until now, but it's important to show your trust (even if your faith is a little shaky) because it will help build your partner's confidence in his or her ability to care for your child. Often, in families where there's a child with an illness or a developmental disorder, one parent takes the lead and the other slinks back, unsure how to respond or afraid that what he or she has to offer isn't good enough. Your partner may come across as being unable to accept a diagnosis or unwilling to participate, when the opposite is true. He or she could simply be overwhelmed.

If after much effort your partner still refuses to accept, or is even hostile about the diagnosis to the point where it's affecting you and hampering your child's progress, you may need to consider more drastic measures. No matter how much you've always loved and respected your spouse, your child needs supportive and attentive parents. Having one of them missing in action can inadvertently sabotage her development, and that is neither fair nor responsible. Your child needs you to be strong and to watch out for her interests. If this is the case, a mediator may help you and your partner come to closure, and perhaps part ways, in a nondestructive fashion.

Sometimes I find myself angry at my child for being autistic. Is this normal?

Anger is a normal reaction under the circumstances. It's human to feel furious at the hand you've been dealt, and you'll be looking for someone on whom to lay the blame. Your expectations are shattered, replaced by a strange existence with which you're unfamiliar, and it looks as if you have no other choice but to accept it.

It's common for parents to feel resentful sometimes at all the extra responsibilities autism places on their shoulders. And since the load is directly connected to your child, you may feel upset with her too, especially on rough days when nothing you try is working at all or your child's symptoms are in high gear. With everything your family's going through, you can't be expected to always be in a good mood. You're allowed the full gamut of emotions: happiness, fear, sadness, anger. That's why it's important to have an outlet that enables you to vent these feelings safely—a daily walk, a journal, a listening ear.

However, it's one thing to be furious about your circumstances, and another to direct the brunt of your frustrations at your child. She is not at fault. She didn't choose to be autistic. She may not even be aware that she has problems that break your heart. Instead, she's going about her days doing what feels most comfortable to her, reacting in the only way she knows. For her to succeed at any of the interventions you choose, she needs your patient hand to guide her.

But everyone has a bad day when you have to struggle mightily for hours over the smallest tasks—getting your child to eat a healthful meal or dress up in clothing that's appropriate for the weather or staying strapped in the car seat. If you're near a boiling point, take deep breaths and a sanity break: Dance around your living room with your child to give yourself an energy boost, or ask your partner to take over and lock yourself in the bathroom for a refreshing, uninterrupted shower.

If at any time you feel as if you may actually act on your anger, or you can't seem to control the mounting fury, situate your child someplace safe in your house and move to another room to clear your thoughts. If you can't calm down, call a trusted friend or family member and ask them to come over and spell you while you get some air. If your anger is all-consuming, seek the help of a therapist or psychologist immediately. You may need to work through your demons with the help of experts who can help you manage your anger. Your child's safety is paramount, and getting help early on is key.

Why did this happen to us?

Rest assured that nearly every person who's been through what you have has probably asked this question at least once. When life throws you a dizzying curve ball, you can lose faith. But know that you did nothing that made your child autistic. She has been given this particular challenge to face, just as other people face challenges of their own, although their particular trial may not be neurological or even physical. With you by her side, and with the assistance of her relatives, friends, doctors, teachers, and therapists, your child will find a way to manage the disorder and all that it brings.

If you find that you're constantly overpowered by feelings of hopelessness, talk to a confidant, counselor or spiritual advisor. He or she can help guide you out of your crisis of faith so you'll feel sufficiently empowered to provide your child with the support required to weather autism's many challenges.

All these appointments with doctors and therapists are wearing me down. How do I juggle everything?

There's one remedy: Get organized. It's the only way you'll stay on top of a hectic schedule filled with lots of comings and goings. A planner in which you can keep track of your appointments will come in handy, as well as an address book or business card holder that can keep important numbers in one place. If you want to opt for something a little more high tech, choose a handheld personal digital assistant (PDA) that can collect your pertinent information in one minuscule gadget. Be sure to pencil in every single meeting; if you use your planner only intermittently, it won't keep you organized at all.

At home, set up in a central location a calendar to which you can transfer information about whatever appointments you've jotted down in your planner every few days. Ask the rest of the family to write down their events, too, so everyone can keep track of each other's schedules. If a conflict arises (say your eldest child has a school performance on the day you've scheduled speech therapy for your younger one), you'll be able to spot it right away and move activities around as you see fit.

Setting up an information system that lays out in detail your upcoming plans is just the first step, however. Keeping all these appointments is another issue altogether. First, learn how to ask for help. You won't be able to do everything alone, especially if you and your spouse both work or have other children. You may be surprised to discover just how many friends and family members are willing to fill in for you when you need assistance. If they offer, take them up on it; if they don't, ask anyway. If you appear at all efficient, others may assume you have everything under control when in reality, you don't.

Be specific about the help you need; for example, ask someone to bring dinner on one hectic night instead of saying "whatever day works for you." Remember, too, that they're doing you a favor, so be sure to take their needs into consideration as well; requesting that a fellow mother who's strapped for time spend two hours calling potential therapists for your child could be too much, but asking her to babysit your other kids while you interview doctors might suit her schedule better. And always say thank you, which is easy to forget when you're struggling to meet so many demands.

Also, take breaks from all the doctor- or therapy-hopping. A diagnosis of autism can be all-consuming; the interventions alone can take up to forty hours a week. But you and your family can't run on empty, so make time for fun. Be sure to take good care of yourself: Eat well, get plenty of rest and exercise to release stress. Rent a family movie, stay in for the night, and ban all talk of autism. Or host a dinner party to thank your helpers but try to avoid making autism the night's topic of conversation. For you to be able to continue helping your child, you need planned breaks from the whirlwind from time to time. When you return to your hectic timetable, you'll be refreshed and ready to take on whatever comes your way.

Why do I sometimes feel that all the work we do to cope is futile?

Many parents just like you find themselves cycling between two distinct emotions—hope and despair. No wonder: Managing autism sometimes feels like taking three steps forward and two steps back; progress can be so incremental it can be hard to measure. Don't be surprised if you find yourself in a "down" phase; it's not easy to stay upbeat all the time, especially when you're fatigued from everything that you need to do to ensure that your child is getting the help she needs.

When you're feeling discouraged, it helps to remind yourself of any successes you've had since you discovered the diagnosis, no matter how small or long ago it's been. If you've only recently learned that your child is autistic, remind yourself how confusing it was months ago when you'd notice your child doing something or acting in a certain manner that you didn't recognize in other children. You may have blamed her for what was happening, or yourself for not knowing just how to parent her. Now, at least, you're aware of what's in store for your family and may already have a plan in place (or at least devising one) to tackle the disorder. That's progress!

If your child has been in an intervention program for some time and seems to be making little headway, know that she's getting the help she needs and that growth and advancement sometimes happens in small steps. What may appear to be hardly a change to others may actually be significant for your child; for example, if at first she used to eat only one or two kinds of food (say, milk and cereal) because of sensory issues and can now ingest the occasional piece of toast, that's a definite improvement.

Sometimes, happiness is all in the way we define progress. Set major milestones and you may not notice the small triumphs along the way that add up to one gigantic stride. Make every single nudge forward count and you'll be able to take pride and joy in how far your child has come.

Where can I find other parents like me?

It's a good instinct to want to seek out other parents who are going through experiences similar to yours, because there's comfort to be found in knowing you're not alone. And thanks to the Internet, it's that much easier to reach out. The Autism Society of America's Web site (www. autism-society.org) is a good place to start; there you will find a list of local chapters and their contact information, including dates when their members get together.

Online support groups abound on the Internet, and many parents of autistic children participate in the forums because it is so easy to do during their downtime. Here are some sites to try:

- The Autism Community Connection (www.autismcommunitycon-nection.com)
- Autism USA (www.autismusa.net)
- BBB Autism (www.bbbautism.com)
- Together for Autism (www.togetherforautism.org)
- Parenting Web sites such as Babycenter.com and Ivillage.com also host bulletin boards for parents of children with disabilities

There are many more. Check the Resources section in the back of this book.

If you much prefer to meet others in person, ask your child's pediatrician or therapist for suggestions on how to network with other parents in your community. Befriend other parents you run into at your child's school or therapy appointments, or start a support group yourself. Post a flyer at your doctor's office to drum up interest; you'll be surprised at how many other moms and dads are aching to share their stories. The Resources section of this book also includes an extensive rundown of organizations across the nation.

5.

TREATMENTS AND INTERVENTIONS

. . . .

Want to know which approach may work best in the management of your child's autism? Read on for insight into the many ways experts teach your child how to gain and master new skills and take charge of their day-to-day challenges.

Why is early intervention important?

Autism experts can't emphasize the value of early intervention in addressing the burgeoning behaviors and symptoms associated with autism. As with many other conditions, be they physical, mental, emotional, or neurological, the earlier the disorder is diagnosed, the better the outcome. That's because you can more successfully find solutions to problems when they're not so ingrained and when the more serious ones have yet to surface.

Research shows that *comprehensive* and *intensive* early intervention makes a big difference in whether autistic children can participate in mainstream classrooms and learn alongside their peers who don't have the disorder. It can also influence the degree of developmental gains kids with ASD will be able to make, including forging relationships with families and friends and acquiring skills they can apply in school as well as in daily life. In some cases, children have improved so much and so quickly that it's hard to tell them apart from those who aren't autistic. They've learned how to manage the disorder and have come to terms with it. But just as important as getting help early is finding the right kind of assistance for your child.

We didn't realize our child was autistic until he was older (age five and up). Will this delayed diagnosis hurt him permanently?

It's unfortunate that your child wasn't discovered to be on the autism spectrum sooner, but there are still many ways he can benefit from various behavioral interventions. You're not alone: Many parents find that before their child is identified as autistic, he has already gone through a battery of tests and labels; but as doctors, therapists, and teachers become more familiar with the disorder, they'll spot it much more quickly, thereby helping many children to receive proper treatment from as early as the toddler years.

The next immediate step in the process is to get your child into some sort of intervention and educational program immediately. The sooner he gets help, the better. It won't help to dwell on what might have been, as that may only compound the frustration you may feel about not having gotten answers earlier on. Nor will it serve any purpose if you blame yourself for the delay in diagnosis. Autism is a difficult disorder to nail down, a fact to which many veteran parents will attest.

Although early diagnosis (age three and younger) is ideal, your child will still be able to make strides and find success if you cobble together a plan that works well for him. He may need a host of therapies and interventions, and may require a more intensive approach, given that he's starting at a later age. This may entail more one-on-one sessions with therapists, more appointments with doctors and psychologists, or simply more of your time. Regimens aimed at younger children may not work well for him, and since he's older, he may have a challenging time adapting to new routines that the interventions you subscribe to may require. It's not easy to predict the outcomes of treatments for autistic children and how they will do over time; but as long as you identify a group of healthcare providers in whom you trust and who are experts in treating children with autism, and you agree with their approach, and your child gets the proper educational and emotional support at school and at home, he's well on his way to becoming his best self.

COMMON TRADITIONAL THERAPIES

What is applied behavior analysis (ABA)?

Applied Behavioral Analysis (ABA) is by far the most common education and intervention plan followed by parents of autistic children. A few variations exist, but the program that's proven popular, known as the UCLA Model of Applied Behavior Analysis, is the brainchild of Dr. O. Ivar Lovaas, the executive director of the Lovaas Institute for Early Intervention in Los Angeles, California. ABA is an approach rooted in the fundamentals of behavior modification, which many psychologists employ in treating all sorts of physical, mental, and emotional disorders.

ABA plays a large role in many educational programs designed especially for autistic children. It's meant to improve communication skills, foster social interaction, encourage play, and help autistic kids become more independent. Vanessa Jenses, executive director of the Cleveland Clinic's Center for Autism, which uses ABA as the foundation for its interventions and strategies, says it does so by using a "systematic application of behavioral treatment" to change the behavior of children with autism and PDD.

ABA practitioners approach their work by understanding that autism is a developmental disorder, one that's biological and neurological in nature and that can be tracked by studying brain functioning and behavior. Autistic children, unlike other kids, aren't "wired" to interpret the world and the people in it as easily or as clearly as the rest of us. A light touch may feel like a shove; basic eye contact may come across as debilitatingly intrusive; a whisper can seem as loud as a sonic boom. Add to these experiences the autistic child's inability to let grown-ups know exactly how they're feeling and filtering all this stimuli, and you have a child who may seem, to those who are uneducated about autism or are unaware the child is autistic, out of control, over-reactive, or cold and distant.

The responses of autistic children are all they know; but these kids can be taught new ways of managing and responding to the world. Through educational methods such as discrete trials, prompting, and reinforcement, kids who follow the ABA program set target goals of behavior and reach them by approaching each new situation with a toolbox of skills they've acquired through repeated practice and drills. ABA professionals work on helping kids to master socially acceptable behaviors and to give up inappropriate ones. Success in one area (eye contact, for example) may lead to attempting even bigger goals (saying "hello" during personal introductions, for one).

What first takes place if you choose to venture down the ABA path is a diagnostic assessment, which examines your child's behavioral issues, how long your child has exhibited them, the reasons to which you attribute these behaviors, and what happens when your child acts in a particular manner.

After this evaluation, your child's ABA therapist, with your input, devises an individualized plan of action and implements it in one-on-one sessions. During these meetings, an effective ABA therapist studies closely the "cause-and-effect" relationships between a situation and your child's reaction. She examines her method as she teaches your child a skill as well as the characteristics of the environment that may have an effect on your child's response, and then tries to accurately measure the effects.

At these sessions, you, as parents, are expected to watch and learn so you can then use the same strategies to help your child on your own; it's important that you're able to implement the same strategies at home. After all, consistency is vital, since varying from the norm may make it difficult for the ABA therapist and you to evaluate what truly works and what doesn't. In between appointments, you may be asked to keep a diary of your child's problematic behaviors (such as banging his head against a wall or scratching your face), noting what may have triggered them, how you responded, and how your child met that response. Parents of children with severe autism often elect to augment the sessions with a formalized home-based program in which they're taught techniques and activities in which they can engage their kids at home. They check in periodically with an ABA center's staff members for feedback and advice, and home visits are scheduled.

Here's a simplified example of what may take place at an ABA one-on-one session: Let's say the ABA therapist is working with a child on completing a simple puzzle. They sit at a table across from each other at eye level. Whereas your child normally throws pieces of a puzzle across the room, during the session they practice putting the pieces of a puzzle together. When the child manages to complete the puzzle on his own, for example, the therapist may give him a piece of fruit, a cookie, a favorite toy, or even a tickle. The therapist then records the child's response. When improvements in behavior appear to be on their way to becoming permanent, the tangible rewards are phased out, replaced by a child's developing ability to discern the pleasing results that their appropriate behavior engenders in others.

Some say ABA is based in part on research by theorist/scientist B.F. Skinner, who found that behavior could be molded through a process called "operant conditioning." In some of his experiments, animals were taught behaviors (e.g., getting a rat to use an automatic food dispenser) that, if mastered, resulted in them getting a reward. While ABA experts don't claim that kids should be trained the same way animals are, children—autistic or not—do learn through repetition, and this is the cornerstone of ABA's philosophy. According to Leslie Sinclair, program director at the Cleveland Clinic's Center for Autism, toddlers do well with intensive, one-on-one therapy. The repetitive nature of ABA drives home its lessons, and as they learn how to behave they can master new skills.

Autistic kids may not easily grasp the concept of learning, but they discover, through the help of their ABA therapist, how to better understand the learning process. In essence, writes Richard Saffran, father of an autistic child and an expert in ABA, they "learn to learn." When one-on-one sessions are over, the regimen is continued at home, tackling more complex skills as the child grows older. Ideally, the treatment plan continues in a classroom that uses ABA as the foundation for the school's educational philosophies.

ABA's biggest asset may be its longevity. Its stature as the most established of treatment strategies for autistic children gives it much-deserved credibility, as do the reams of data and studies that have shown its success in helping kids function happily and well in society. In 1987, Lovaas published groundbreaking research that showed that the drills that make up a large portion of the ABA method were successful in helping autistic children, some of whom exhibited such great gains that they no longer appeared to be on the spectrum. Autism expert Richard L. Simpson, writing in the summer 2001 issue of the journal *Focus on Autism and Other Developmental Disabilities,* observed that there is "overwhelming evidence that methods based on the behaviorally based principles of ABA form the foundation of many effective individualized programs and generally bode well for achievement of desired outcomes among individuals with autism spectrum disorders." In plain English, ABA works for lots of autistic kids. And ABA proponents have tons of research to prove it.

Another reason autistic children who follow ABA are successful is the program's emphasis on one-on-one instruction, at least in the initial stages. With such close study, an ABA therapist can keep a watchful eye on what's working and what's not, and tailor the sessions accordingly. Although it's not required of a successful regimen, one-on-one sessions ensure your child gets a great deal of individualized attention.

Even though children in ABA environments participate in drills, and they're expected to learn a set of skills—a "curriculum" of sorts—these sessions cannot, by any means, be described as cookie-cutter. Instead, you and your therapist work together to come up with the best strategy, using the science of ABA, for your child.

Does ABA have any shortcomings?

Like any other approach, ABA doesn't work for every child. One of the biggest disadvantages of committing to a true ABA treatment plan (one that includes extensive one-on-one sessions and evaluations, training, and materials) is how much you could end up paying for it. Plainly put, ABA can be prohibitively expensive. It can cost as much as, if not more than, tuition at a top-notch private elementary school, running in the tens of thousands of dollars each year. Fees covering ten months of training at the

Princeton Child Development Institute in New Jersey, a nationally re-nowned research, treatment, and ABA-based educational center for autistic children, total more than $45,000, wrote Iver Peterson in a May 2000 front-page story in *The New York Times*. A portion of the expenses may be covered by insurance, but most parents eke out a way to pay out of pocket. Learning ABA methods and then opting for a home-based approach is one way to cut the costs, but studies show that children are likelier to thrive in an ABA classroom or one-on-one environment.

Some parents gripe that ABA is far too rigid and that "training" children feels "unnatural" or "forced." They complain that the technique of repetition teaches autistic kids only to respond to specific cues, and doesn't help them change their approach to events in everyday life. They use the old argument that it's like giving a man a fish so he can eat for one day instead of teaching him how to fish so he'll learn how to eat for the rest of his life.

But as with the other interventions, it matters where you go for help and whom you consult. An institution may claim to subscribe to the ABA method, but may not train its teachers adequately in it so they can actually make a difference in the lives of their young clients.

In his *Times* article, Peterson described ABA as "very expensive . . . coaching." Kathy Mannion, executive director for the Association for Science in Autism Treatment immediately objected to that notion, expressing her dissent in a letter to the *Times* editor in which she asserted that ABA is "the only treatment intervention for autism that has withstood scientific scrutiny for more than thirty years." In many cases, parents sign up for the classes, and as they master the techniques themselves, discontinue training (thereby saving money) and apply what they learn at home until it's almost second nature.

What is the Developmental, Individual Difference Relationship–Based Model (DIR/Floortime)?

Grown-ups may have their jobs, but for kids, their life's work is play. Children learn and grow when they indulge in play, but for children with autism, play may represent a way out of their enclosed world. That's the thinking behind the Developmental, Individual Difference Relationship–Based Model (DIR Model), also known as "Floortime."

This method was conceived by Dr. Stanley Greenspan, a child psychiatrist and professor of psychiatry, behavioral sciences, and pediatrics at George Washington University Medical School. In his book *The Child with Special Needs,* he outlines a way for young children to be evaluated for developmental disorders such as autism and PDD by checking if they've reached six crucial milestones: (1) showing interest in the "sights, sounds, and sensations of the world" and the ability to soothe oneself when upset; (2) relating with others; (3) displaying the ability to "engage in two-way communication with gestures"; (4) creating "complex gestures, to string together a series of actions into an elaborate and deliberate problem-solving experience"; (5) discerning and grasping concepts; and (6) making connections between ideas and implementing these connections into their daily lives.

Compared to other children, autistic kids have difficulty reaching some or all of these milestones. Some fail to reach them altogether. For example, a child with autism or PDD may be able to pick up a block and hold it, but won't stack a few of them to make a tower. Or he may not know how to tell you he wants milk instead of juice, and instead grunts or flails on the floor. He can't communicate his needs (which he may be unable to identify) with his parents, and both sides end up frustrated.

Through his work as a developmental psychiatrist, Greenspan discovered that children grasp ideas through emotions. If autistic children don't know what it is they feel, or if they can somewhat identify their emotions but don't know how to process them, they're challenged when facing a simple task that nonautistic kids learn to perform with ease: understanding life and the world beyond the literal. But there's more. If children have physical or biological problems that make it more difficult for them to tune into their emotions (which autistic children often do, in the form of sensory overload, the coordination issues, or the inability to recognize their own space and the way their bodies move in it), then they are hampered even further. They have to jump through yet another hoop on their way to developmental progress.

Greenspan's theory was revolutionary. The idea that tuning into feelings and emotions and learning empathy were so instrumental in brain development initially placed him at odds with the generally accepted approach to treating autism at the time, which favored the behavior modification route. But soon his novel ideas won over professionals in the field of autism and pediatrics. Now Greenspan's theory is the basis for a few popular offshoots of Floortime, such as the PLAY Project (Play and Language for Autistic Youngsters), an autism intervention program run by Dr. Rick Solomon, clinical associate professor at the University of Michigan's Department of Pediatrics.

So what is Floortime and how can it help? Floortime encourages parents and caregivers to open and close "circles of communication" with autistic kids. A circle is opened when you engage your child in a form of dialogue or interaction (for example, you tap your child's nose playfully) and is closed, or completed, when he responds (perhaps he'll tap your nose in return). As more and more circles are opened and closed between you and your child, your bond strengthens, trust increases, and in that environment, learning can take place.

To this end, Floortime (and other Floortime-based programs) advocates intensive sessions (up to 20–40 hours a week) that begin as one-on-one interactions (so as not to overwhelm the child) but may progress to a group environment. The goal is for your autistic child to move up through six "functional developmental levels" (FDLs): engagement and shared attention (FDLs 1 and 2); two-way communication (FDLs 3 and 4); shared meanings and symbolic play (FDL 5); and emotional thinking (FDL 6). At the same time, your child will also work with speech and occupational therapists and other healthcare providers who will address his other needs. If he also has a hearing problem, for example, part of his "team" will be his audiologist.

The first session comprises an evaluation performed usually at the Floortime specialist's clinic; at the PLAY Project, for example, children are assessed by Dr. Solomon during a comprehensive review, at which a diagnosis of autism is confirmed (or, in some cases, given for the first time). Ten to twelve visits with a PLAY consultant follow in your home, where he or she will teach you how to play with toys and prompt your child in a way that opens and closes those crucial circles. Sessions are done at home because that's where your child is most comfortable, theoretically, and his props will be the toys he's used to working with every day. (You can choose to augment your child's toy chest with new playthings that may elicit more of a response, but the basic concept behind PLAY is that anything can be made into a toy to draw your child out of his autistic world. A salt shaker or a light switch, for example, can provide moments of wonder.)

Often misunderstood, Floortime isn't just about sitting down and playing in the same fashion you play with your children normally. It's about playing with them in a way that helps them make connections, not only with the toy or with the rules of a game, but with you. Patricia Stacey, mother of Walker, a seven-year-old boy who first started working with Greenspan in 1996 when Walker was barely a year old, has recounted her experiences in her memoir, *The Boy Who Liked Windows.* "Greenspan told us that we would need to make Walker work for what he wanted," writes Stacey. "That every desire would be satisfied through human interaction." The Floortime "play dates" are meant to be animated; the livelier you are, the likelier you'll be able to entice your child to respond.

More important, although you're facilitating the play, it's your child who leads the sessions, not you. Floortime prides itself on being "child-centered," which means these "intensive socialization" sessions will be made up of games your child wants to play in the manner in which he wants to play them. If he's enamored of trains, you'll likely be spending lots of time with trains until he shows interest in other things. But there are myriad ways to play with trains other than leading them on tracks. Your train may one day fly, or hop like a kangaroo, or do whatever it is your child wants it to.

All that one-on-one fun time seems to work, too. According to an article on the PLAY Project in the fall 2002 issue of *Medicine at Michigan,* a

2001 National Academy of Sciences report "backs this premise, recommending that young children with autism receive at least twenty-five hours per week of intensive socialization, language, and academic work, in a low adult-child ratio."

One of Floortime's biggest draws is the way it empowers parents, giving them control over their children's treatment and an active role in encouraging their development. While it requires a few initial training sessions conducted by a Floortime professional, you are quickly shepherded into position as your child's primary therapist. Considering that one of the first signs parents report to doctors when they suspect their child has autism is his or her lack of connection with them—a take-my-parents-or-leave-them attitude, if you will—being able to bond and interact with their child, to be able to reach them on an emotional level, is powerful. Parents often say this is one of the greatest gifts of Floortime; it's good that their children can now say a dozen words, but more important is that they can also give and receive hugs, they can acknowledge their parents' existence, and they exhibit an attachment to their parents that wasn't present before.

"Floortime is our time together," says Carol Thomas of Lansing, Michigan, mother of Jacob and Joshua, four-year-old twins she's raising with her partner, Mabel. "I get to do it, not some therapist at a clinic where I drop them off. It's wonderful to be able to help your own child improve and learn new skills. And besides, I know them best."

Patricia Stacey echoes this same sense of autonomy. She writes, "A therapist alone couldn't teach an autistic child to come out of his world; the parents (or someone else with an emotional connection to the child) would have to be involved. The foundation of cognitive development would need to be laid at home."

Floortime is also affordable. Training sessions may cost anywhere from a few hundred to a few thousand dollars, but after the initial outlay, expenses can be kept to a minimum. While you'll probably want to stock up your toy chest at home and replenish the supply with more interesting playthings once or twice a year, you're not expected to purchase expensive toys or prescribed kits for learning. Nearly anything, as long as it's child-safe and kid-friendly, can be used as a jumping-off point for making connections and creating those proverbial "circles."

Are there disadvantages to Floortime?

What makes Floortime so attractive to some parents may be the same reason it doesn't work for others—many value its flexible structure, but others feel it's too open-ended, not goal-oriented enough. When Sarah, the daughter of Canton, Michigan, mom Jill Gregory, was diagnosed with autism at age three, Gregory and her husband shopped around for an intervention that would work best for Sarah and the rest of the family. The couple vacillated between ABA and Floortime for months, and even hired therapists from both camps for preliminary trial runs, but in the end, the Gregorys decided on a program that was based heavily on ABA.

"My husband liked the fact that Sarah's progress was measurable with ABA," says Gregory in an interview. "You set short goals and can check them off on a mental list. It was therapeutic for us, too, to be able to see how she was improving from week to week or month to month."

Gregory goes on to comment that while she appreciated and supported the ideas on which Floortime is founded—engaging the child and creating circles of communication that grow larger and more complex over time—she and her spouse doubted it would work for Sarah, who was diagnosed with moderate-to-severe autism and was completely nonverbal and unresponsive. "To try to get into her world and create 'circles,' as Floortime would have us do, was incredibly difficult," she says. "If I sat down to play with her, she'd get up and leave. We had to do something more in-your-face, more intensive."

Even after having been implemented for decades by Dr. Greenspan and other autism experts, Floortime is still a relative newcomer when compared to ABA; it doesn't boast as many studies to support its findings. However, it appears to have garnered praise, enough to be combined with ABA in some programs, and scores of satisfied parents testify that it can work with their children. (Recent statistics compiled by the DIR-based PLAY Project, found that "a study of 200 children clearly diagnosed with autism, with a follow-up greater than or equal to two years, showed 58 percent had a good to outstanding outcome.")

Can we subscribe to simultaneous multiple interventions—ABA *and* Floortime, for example?

Many families subscribe to one approach and commit to it completely because they find it's easier to do so. And if the intervention they've chosen appears to be working, understandably they feel reluctant to fix what isn't essentially "broke." But many other families have found that an interdisciplinary approach is more effective. They gather a set of tools to work with and commit to whatever seems to work best depending on which sort of problem their child is trying to master. Some autism researchers agree, saying there's value in mixing and matching. "In the absence of reliable scientific evidence regarding exclusive and extensive use of any intervention method, including ABA, it is prudent to individualize strategies to fit children and families," Richard L. Simpson writes in the summer 2001 issue of *Focus on Autism and Other Developmental Disabilities*. "Exclusive use of any program may be appropriate for some students, families, and professionals but clearly would not be the preferred intervention under every condition for all."

COMMON SUPPLEMENTARY REGIMENS

What is sensory integration therapy?

Many children on the spectrum suffer from sensory dysfunction, meaning any or all of their five senses aren't able to take in the information they're supposed to accept and process in order to understand what they're seeing, hearing, tasting, feeling, or smelling. They may suffer from too much stimulation from the sensory input or hardly register it at all. Imagine feeling assaulted by everything that comes your way, either through sight, sound, or any of the other senses; you'd scarcely be able to concentrate on the task at hand or even function. No wonder autistic children flap their hands, squeal, or cover their ears—perhaps they're merely trying to cope in an overstimulating world. On the other hand, imagine what it would be like in a world where you can barely feel the touch of a hand against your skin, or discern noises projected at conversational levels. The world would be a silent place and you wouldn't feel motivated to reach out. Whatever kind of sensory integration issues a child with ASD has, you can bet he's working with a deficit, as our senses provide our brains with the valuable data we need to move about in this world. When these senses are not working properly, a child is at a disadvantage.

The primary goal of sensory integration therapy is to help a child learn how to find equilibrium in three areas: the tactile system (sense of touch); vestibular system (which affects one's ability to gauge one's space and how to move in it); and the proprioceptive system (the area that handles motor skills). Sensory integration therapists aim to help children balance the input they receive so they can learn and respond to the stimuli accordingly.

In early sessions, a therapist evaluates a child's reactions to sensory stimuli. The information gathered is then used to create a personalized regimen— a "diet" of sorts—which works on the child's skills that need improvement. For example, if your child hates to touch soft, "squishy" things, the therapist can help the child overcome this aversion by slowly introducing items made of foam or putty during sessions and letting the youngster handle them when ready and willing. If the child has problems balancing, a therapist may put him or her on swings or balance beams to help work on equilibrium.

For more information on sensory integration issues, see Chapter 3: Manifestations.

What is TEACCH?

Created by Eric Schopler in 1972, TEACCH (Treatment and Education of Autistic and related Communication handicapped CHildren), known more accurately as Division TEACCH, is a community-based program that incorporates a handful of systems and approaches to help an autistic individual learn and become a respected and valuable member of society. It isn't so much a regimen as a service, an almost one-stop-shop organization that provides a wide range of services, from diagnostic help to interventions. It was established in North Carolina and is headquartered at the University of North Carolina at Chapel Hill's Department of Psychiatry. It has been so successful that the state legislature mandated its existence and the entire state subscribes to the program. It may actually be the program with the most reach in any given locale. Many community autism programs in other states have used TEACCH as a model, but for now the program itself is only used in North Carolina.

Residents of North Carolina who are autistic receive aid through the organizing body, and it has served as a model for programs that may be implemented nationally and abroad in the near future. So impressive is its impact that TEACCH is now held up as the standard by many experts. International professionals involved in the autism community, from Iceland to Hong Kong, have attended its training courses.

Within North Carolina, the program offers parents one organization to contact for help, minimizing confusion and giving them a central resource to consult. Think your child is autistic but don't know how to proceed from there? Contact TEACCH. Not sure how to implement a workable system at home so that your child can concentrate on mastering skills? TEACCH can guide you. Don't quite know how to handle the strains of parenting an autistic child? TEACCH will assist in finding you the help to work through your emotions.

TEACCH recommends a great deal of structure within an autistic person's environment, including thoughtfully designed study and play areas, schedules and lessons, and focuses on clear communication. It relies heavily on visuals, using them as prompts or reminders to help participants understand what's happening and what is expected of them in a given situation. In a nod to sensory integration techniques, it also takes into account that many autistic children suffer from stimulatory overload, and works to accommodate them. It also helps parents of autistic children and their caretakers understand that not all characteristics of the developmental disorder are to be perceived as drawbacks; in fact, proponents of TEACCH take advantage of, among many other skills, the intense ability to focus and memorize that many autistic kids display. What others may consider weaknesses are seen as strengths on which to build even more mastery. The end goal: to ensure that those living with the disorder not be institutionalized and that they acquire the necessary know-how to be able to participate in, and contribute to, their local community.

EDUCATIONAL SUPPLEMENTS/TOOLS

What are social stories?

Educator Carol Gray, who runs the Gray Center for Social Learning and Understanding in Jenison, Michigan, came up with the concept of "social stories" as a way to teach individuals with ASD about ways to behave in various social situations, scenarios that are very difficult for those with the disorder. Because so much of social interaction depends on being able to read others and react to their emotional cues, a skill that's challenging for even the highest functioning, Gray's social stories provide autistic children with a blueprint for what's expected in various circumstances. Social stories have a specific format—they are fairly short, present an idea or a situation, describe that situation's possible outcome, and then teach a lesson in a way that individuals with ASD will understand. The stories are usually written in the first person, and are generally upbeat in nature. They're not meant to relay punishment for untoward behaviors, but instead teach alternative responses. Even the way a social story is disseminated is carefully thought out; they're taught in a soothing and non-jarring manner and require a straightforward and patient attitude on the part of the storyteller. The Gray Center makes available books and videos on how to create a social story that's appropriate and effective for individuals with ASD and can also provide training for those seeking to master the system more thoroughly.

What is a visual schedule?

Visual schedules help autistic individuals understand what happens and how to behave during a specific event in their daily life or throughout the routine of a whole day. For example, through a series of pictures or illustrations your child can learn what actions will take place during a trip to a grocery store. Illustrations would show the car that you take to get there, the store itself, the grocery cart, some typical items you buy, the checkout counter, among others. Also, a teacher, parent, or caregiver can outline a sequence of events for the day. Pictures could include a table with a cereal bowl on top to signify breakfast, a sink to show how to clean the dishes, a closet to remind the child to get dressed, a teacher to indicate that the youngster needs to go to school, and so on. When explaining the schedule to your child, words like "first," "next," and "then" are usually given as verbal sequencing cues.

Verbal schedules are helpful to autistic children because the youngsters aren't always able to grasp the concept of time and often have trouble adjusting from one activity to the next. Given fair warning with the help of a visual schedule, autistic children are able to anticipate changes and can manage transitions more smoothly.

What is an object exchange?

Object exchange is a system that some parents and caregivers of autistic children employ to facilitate communication. If your child is extremely nonverbal, this may be effective for you. Essentially, it works this way: You teach your child that an object, say, a ball, symbolizes "playtime." If you want him to let you know that he wants to participate in a game, you demonstrate for him that giving you the ball initiates that activity. If he wants to eat a cookie, he can hand you a plate. Object exchange instructs your child in the rudiments of cause and effect, which PECS (see below) and other educational systems also do. When he masters this give-and-take, he'll be able to anticipate that providing you with an item will make happen something he wants to happen.

What are PECS?

Developed to help children and adults with disabilities, especially those who have trouble speaking, the Picture Exchange Communication System (PECS) uses reinforcement as a way to help people learn how to communicate. This therapy is a nod to the tenets of Applied Behavior Analysis (ABA). Teachers using PECS, who also call themselves "trainers," must first identify what it is that would motivate a child to learn. After they figure out what a specific student likes and will respond to, they use that object as a way to reward a child who grasps the basic communication exchange in which they're trying to instruct him. Other fundamental tools are pictures of the rewards that allow an autistic child to let the person with whom he's trying to "talk" know what it is he wants.

One of the first lessons trainers usually try to impart is how to ask for something or request an activity. A PECS teacher, after choosing a reward based on the child with whom she's interacting, will then show the reward to the child and when he grabs for it, he's shown a picture that communicates what he needs. He is taught to pick up the picture and give it to the teacher in order to receive the reward. When he has received the reward, which is also labeled, he will learn to identify the objects by their names. For example, say a child is obsessed with cars, a Matchbox truck would be an appropriate and effective reward. When a child manages to give a picture of a car to the teacher, then the teacher hands him the toy vehicle.

As a child masters one mode of communication, he is eased into more sophisticated exchanges. Later, he may be able to use a card to let someone know what he's feeling or thinking about an event that's taking place. Instead of making a simple request, the autistic child is now communicating ideas.

Do medications for autistic children work?

In some cases, medication may be warranted for your child, and indeed, some varieties appear to hold promise for autistic individuals. Most classes of drugs address one type of behavior associated with autism, and few of them are meant to minimize all behavioral and emotional problems. Parents and doctors who opt for medication sometimes choose a combination of drugs to provide the best possible treatment. The following are the types of drugs commonly prescribed:

- Antidepressants classified as selective serotonin reuptake inhibitors, SSRIs, are often relied upon to reduce obsessive or self-destructive behaviors seen in some children with autism. They work by altering brain chemistry by influencing the levels of serotonin. Sample brand names include Prozac, Paxil, Celexa, and Zoloft. Many therapists are encouraged by the beneficial effects of SSRIs—their effects on autism have been documented through some reputable studies—but others worry about the dangers of providing young children with powerful drugs generally prescribed for adults. Some of these medications (Paxil, for one) have been associated with a slight increase in suicide among the general teenage population (although recent research disputes this finding). Careful assessment and follow-up by a trained psychiatrist helps ensure they're prescribed and taken appropriately.
- Neuroleptics, sometimes described as tranquilizers, adjust dopamine and serotonin levels in the brain. Risperdal and Zyprexa are two commonly prescribed brands, and appear to lessen moments of extreme aggression in children with autism, in part by sedating them. Use of this class of drugs may affect a child's level of alertness and appetite and cause side effects such as nausea and dizziness. In some cases, they may even trigger problems with regulating blood pressure.
- Anti-seizure medications, under such brand names as Depakote and Neurontine, also mitigate hurtful or injurious behavior in autistic children, as well as explosive moments of rage. They're meant to have

an effect on the area of the brain that controls actions, but have been known to cause liver damage and other serious conditions.

Aside from these major categories, autistic children have also been put on a drug cocktail that includes medications that address their gastrointestinal issues or doses of nicotine to help neuroleptics work more effectively. Although many doctors would agree that medications have a place in the overall treatment of autistic children, some detractors worry that kids are being sedated because it's an easier way to control the less palatable or manageable symptoms of the developmental disorder compared to some of the more proven behavior modification intervention programs that require more attention and help from parents.

Debate continues over just how big a role medications should play in the overall treatment plan for autistic individuals. Noted autism expert Temple Grandin, who lives with the disorder herself, has addressed the issue, acknowledging that some drugs have been shown to be helpful but urging doctors to consider smaller doses, as people with ASD may be more sensitive to medications than others. Some families worry over possible side effects, some of which seem just as injurious as the disorder itself.

Doctors, teachers, and therapists can work with you to evaluate whether or not your child is a good candidate for medications. Ultimately, however, the choice is up to you if your child is a minor; weigh all the benefits and risks so you can arrive at a decision about which you can be confident. Know, too, that drugs can sometimes take time to kick in. You may not be able to see a change overnight, but in time, you'll likely observe some changes, hopefully for the better.

ALTERNATIVE THERAPIES

What is the Son-Rise Program?

The Son-Rise Program is the intervention of choice at the Autism Treatment Center of America, based in Sheffield, Massachusetts. It was conceptualized by Barry Neil Kaufman and Samahria Lyte Kaufman, whose child was diagnosed as autistic, and is an intensive type of treatment that has recently piqued the interest of many parents. Son-Rise is founded on the belief of "love and acceptance," meaning that parents embrace their children's autism and its attendant symptoms and use them to find a way into the autistic youngster's world. Parents are trained in the approach and become the primary therapists, with the home as the center of treatment.

Priding itself as a compassionate form of intervention, the Son-Rise Program believes that parents can reach their children and help them grow and develop by respecting their individuality and by making bonding through interactive play the top priority. Parents are encouraged to display lots of enthusiasm for any activity that holds their kid's attention and to channel that excitement into helping them master new skills. Teachers of this program also believe that when parents follow the lead of a child—a specific technique they call "joining"—when their children exhibit adverse behaviors such as perseveration and stimming, they may actually cause their children to lose interest in those activities.

What is hippotherapy?

Hippotherapy refers to therapeutic horseback riding (as opposed to riding a hippopotamus, as its name may imply), an activity that has proven to be beneficial to children with many disabilities, not just autism. Most children with autism are burdened with many other physical, emotional, and mental problems that necessitate therapies beyond those that address the developmental disorder. And hippotherapy is fast becoming one of the most effective—and entertaining—methods to address those concerns. Physical, speech, and occupational therapists have increasingly been incorporating it into their work, and they now count as some of the biggest proponents of the regimen.

Because it's still a fairly new program for autistic kids, not much has been documented about how it helps them directly. But parents are discovering that their children look forward to time with their horse, appear to come out of their shell during the sessions, and improve various skills. Over the course of a few weeks, a child is introduced to his horse and gets to know her, building trust with the animal and creating a comfortable rapport. Over time, the young rider gets to mount the horse and engages in a series of activities meant to exercise and challenge the five senses. Therapists tailor their sessions to the goals designed for a child—if a rider has problems with coordination and movement, for example, the session is geared toward those concerns. The focus isn't on teaching a child how to ride a horse; instead, the animal is used as a helper while the therapist and the child work on sensory and neurological challenges. According to the American Hippotherapy Association, the activity is especially suited for children who have abnormal muscle tone; impaired balance, coordination, communication, and sensorimotor functions; problems with posture; limited mobility and limb functions; and speech, behavior, cognitive, and gross motor skills issues.

Horses work well with children because they're fairly gentle (especially the ones employed specifically for hippotherapy), provide a warm and soothing presence, and interact well with human beings. In fact, some people think of them as extra-large dogs. And when a child rides a horse, the rhythm mimics that of walking, triggering various sensory and neurological responses. Before your child embarks on a riding program, however, obtain clearance from his pediatrician. You may also want to look into the specific programs you're considering to ascertain their reputability and experience in assisting children who are autistic (they should be aware of all the issues involved). In some cases, hippotherapy qualifies as physical or occupational therapy for insurance purposes, and fees may be partially covered. Check with your insurance provider for more information before you commit to any sessions so you're aware of the cost involved.

What is martial arts therapy?

Therapies that employ one of the martial arts—be it karate, tae kwon do, or any other discipline—have won the support of many parents of autistic children simply because they seem to help. No wonder: Martial arts are meant to build discipline, focus, and self-esteem, goals that would help any child, whether stricken with autism or not. Plus, if your child has problems with coordination and balance or with processing sensory input, martial arts therapies address those concerns as well. Much will depend, though, on how your child is able to function within group settings; some autistic children want nothing to do with crowds and loud noises, both of which are plentiful in a martial arts class. Others will welcome the opportunity to move their body, to mix it up with other kids and expend energy.

As with other therapies, check to make sure the martial arts studio you're considering—often referred to as a dojo—has a program specifically for children with developmental disorders. If ASD children are usually mixed in with typical kids, speak with the instructor to assess whether she's familiar and experienced with dealing with autistic children. Observing a few sessions will give you information on how the instructor runs a class and encourages the children to participate; if you like her style and think it'll mesh well with your child's personality, you may want to test the waters with a class or two.

What is auditory integration therapy?

Many autistic kids are unable to process all the sounds they hear; some noises are pleasant and others come across as overbearing and unmanageable. At times, children are unable to discern one sound from the other, and everything sounds like one cacophonous roar. Or they can make out sounds in one frequency range but not another. Whatever the circumstance, some experts believe autistic kids have the ability to filter out the sounds they don't have the capacity to deal with, and this tendency exacerbates a behavior that many consider "walling out." A child will act as if he can't hear anything and doesn't respond.

Auditory integration therapy (AIT) has made believers out of many parents of autistic children, notably those with speech and hearing problems. These parents report a marked improvement in learning and behavior when their kids go through AIT. They also say their kids seem to better understand what their parents are saying, and tune them out less often. During therapy, an autistic individual learns to distinguish sounds of vari-

ous frequencies because they receive auditory input in ways they can't predict; they sit and listen through headphones but can't anticipate if the next
noise is something they'll want to tune out or something they find easy to
listen to; consequently, they learn to process all incoming input.

What is the gluten-free-casein-free diet? Should I put my child on it?

The gluten-free-casein-free diet (GFCF) severely limits or eliminates from
an autistic child's diet any food items that contain two kinds of protein,
gluten (derived from wheat and other grain products) and casein (which
comes from dairy items). The thinking is that many kids with the developmental disorder have what some experts have described as a "leaky gut,"
which means the intestinal lining is damaged and punctured with minute
openings that prevent it from properly doing its job—processing ingested
food. Others think of it as an allergy. When a child eats food with gluten
and casein, the nutrients apparently break down into peptides that seep
through the openings in the intestines into the bloodstream, causing discomfort in the individual and triggering behavioral problems. Some studies have supported this idea, showing that a number of autistic children
have abnormally elevated amounts of peptides in their urine.

On the face of it, it makes sense that when an autistic child is made to
feel comfortable—in this case, if he's truly allergic to gluten and casein,
when his diet is rid of the offenders—behavioral episodes in which he
"acts out" will diminish. After all, when a person isn't feeling well, he's not
able to function at his best. However, although some parents report that
their child showed progress in behavior and development when put on the
GFCF diet, its effectiveness as a treatment for all autistic children is, according to a study published in a 2000 issue of the journal *Neurology,*
largely unproven. In short, it's hit-or-miss.

So what would be the harm in trying out the GFCF diet? Lots. Re-
moving gluten and casein from everything your child eats is a major task.
If you do so, you'll be drastically calibrating his diet and he won't be

able to eat many kinds of food. Not only will this severely reduce your options—an extreme move considering that many autistic children, especially those with sensory issues, already can't or won't try many different kinds of foods—it may cause your child to develop nutritional deficiencies that can't and shouldn't be countermeasured by administering vitamins. A growing child needs a wide variety of foods to grow healthy and strong, and nutritionists generally frown on diets, especially those for kids, that reduce the intake of vital nutrients and entire food groups. Carbohydrates, the main supply of gluten, are essential for energy and help the brain function well. Dairy products are the best sources of calcium, which promotes bone health. Eliminating food groups, especially in children's diets, is less than ideal; in fact, even followers of the GFCF diet recommend a slow withdrawal of these foods. Making your child go cold turkey might cause extreme swings in his behavior.

If you're interested in the GFCF diet, we suggest you consult a gastroenterologist, food allergist, and dietitian. It makes sense, after all, to have a professional confirm that your child has an aversion to gluten and casein before you go through the trouble of signing up for the diet and instituting it. Many digestive issues and allergies are self-diagnosed, meaning the analysis isn't derived from any medical information. Actually, they're not all that common, in spite of what you may have read or heard. Verifying that your child has this allergy takes more than trial-and-error; that is, you can't just eliminate a food item from his diet, observe his behavior, and then attribute any improvements to the removal of said item. Many other forces affect behavior. Food products rarely boast only one ingredient, and include many other substances that could be the ones your child can't tolerate. Working with a healthcare professional who's expert in the field will ensure that you have the most accurate data before you make a decision about what your child can and can't eat. The GFCF diet is a big step, and it isn't easy to put into practice.

Know, though, that getting tested for allergies may not be a comfortable process for your child; it can entail lengthy and prolonged testing that he may not want to sit through or won't be able to tolerate. Ask your pediatrician or gastroenterologist for help in making any procedure more palatable for your child.

What is chelation and does it work?

Chelation, also known as chelation therapy, is an alternative and controversial method that some practitioners have used to treat children and adults with autism. Various types of medication are introduced into the bloodstream intravenously (through a needle) over a series of appointments, although in some cases, they can also be given orally.

Most proponents of chelation therapy generally subscribe to the theory that mercury poisoning may be the reason a child develops autism; the source of mercury is believed to be primarily from vaccines that contain thimerosal. The human body can't tolerate large amounts of mercury, and chelation therapists argue that children who have been unwittingly exposed to too much of the substance suffer neurological damage, hence the developmental delays and other symptoms.

Before it began to be applied to autism, chelation therapy was successfully used in treating lead poisoning. It has also been employed in the treatment of people who suffer from heart ailments such as atherosclerosis, as well as Parkinson's disease and Alzheimer's, but its effectiveness and safety are still under scrutiny.

The therapy's value in treating children with autism is also heavily debated. Those who believe it's the next biggest cure swear that they see improvements in behavior and learning after their kids have gone through the dozens of infusions required by the regimen. Yet many others, including leading scientists who have researched the disease for years, doubt that it actually accomplishes what it claims.

These experts cite chelation therapy's many dangers and caution parents against committing to this type of unproven regimen for many reasons. First, whether thimerosal-containing vaccines, or vaccines in general, cause autism is still a looming question. Most studies that have looked into the matter found no basis for that conclusion. Therefore, why subject your child to a self-proclaimed "cure" when the reasoning behind it may be fundamentally faulty? Second, there is no true governing body that ensures that chelation therapists are fully schooled in all the risks and issues associated with it. You won't really know, until it may be too late, whether the person you've chosen to chelate your child is a bona fide professional who won't harm him inadvertently. Third, the procedures are prohibitively expensive, sometimes costing hundreds of dollars per session, with dozens of sessions required. Fourth, chelation therapy can have long-lasting, adverse side effects, including kidney damage and congestive heart failure. Last, although some experts claim chelation therapy is safe for kids, it's difficult to know with certainty that your child will not be in danger. Adults need to be comprehensively screened before they can be cleared for treatment, and children are far more vulnerable than their grown-up counterparts. Some parents, in the hope of chancing upon a cure for their child, unfortunately may be putting them in harm's way.

Autism is heartbreaking, not only for the children and adults affected, but for those who love and care for them every day. And it's disheartening to hear that there's no known solution for this growing problem. That's why it's important to exercise scrupulous judgment when evaluating treatments, especially ones like chelation therapy that cause deep dissent among autism experts. Although it's not fair to assume that proponents or practitioners of chelation are merely out to make a quick buck at the expense of desperate parents—some chelation therapists truly believe it's the way to help hundreds of patients with the disorder—there are those who may not hold the best intentions and may not have the background required to provide the service. Ask your child's pediatrician and therapists what their opinion is of chelation, and base your decisions not only on anecdotal evidence but on actual controlled studies that look clearly at the benefits and the dangers. Rather than pursue this route, you may find that you'd rather invest in interventions that involve fewer risks and are backed by science. It can only help your child for you to be a thorough investigator in your quest to find the best way to help him.

What is secretin therapy and is it promising?

Secretin is a hormone produced by the small intestines that helps the pancreas function well during the digestive process. Some people, however, including a number of autistic children, have trouble producing the hormone. Small doses of a synthetic version, derived from a similar hormone found in pigs, is injected in patients while undergoing gastrointestinal procedures such as endoscopies. It's during one of these procedures in 1996 that a New Hampshire couple, Gary and Victoria Beck, is said to have stumbled upon a therapy that made a big difference for their son, Parker.

A few days after their usually nonresponsive autistic son underwent an endoscopy for chronic diarrhea, the Becks were astonished by a marked improvement in his behavior. He started interacting with them, showed interest in his surroundings, and even spoke. When the Becks began retracing their steps to look for the trigger, the only thing they could come up with that diverted from their normal routine was the endoscopy. After asking around, they learned that secretin was injected into their son, and this discovery set them on a mission to prove that secretin could be a potent treatment for autism, even though secretin isn't government-approved for use as medication.

Although the Becks had to search far and wide to find a physician who was willing to work with them and to give Parker secretin every couple of weeks, the Becks believed in the power of the hormone so fully that they were, in effect, testing out an unproven drug. When word got out about its "miraculous" abilities, secretin became the buzzword among many parents of autistic children who were open to trying new therapies. Even the media jumped on the bandwagon, and secretin was featured in television news magazines and in printed media.

Secretin appears to show promise. But unfortunately, as with other "trendy" cures that have come before it, secretin also appears to be undependable at best. For every Parker Beck there are numerous autistic kids for whom secretin has had no effect. Many families were met with disappointment upon finding out that their children didn't respond to the drug. Clinical trials, spurred in part by publicity surrounding the few children who claimed to have experienced marked improvements after using secretin, ended up proving that the drug was no better than other alternative therapies that were first lauded and later disproved. In January 2004, one laboratory, Repligen, which was conducting its own experiments on the drug with the help of 132 young participants, publicly admitted that secretin appeared to have no better effect than a placebo in improving behavior in autistic children. The tests revealed that secretin wasn't the wonder drug many thought it would turn out to be.

Still, there are many who still hope that secretin will prove to be beneficial in the treatment of autistic kids, in spite of numerous signs that suggest otherwise. Although it's difficult to dispute that there have been success stories, there have also been numerous failures; scientists who had been willing to examine the issue came to find no reason to recommend it. Furthermore, secretin is only approved by the Food and Drug Administration for use in small doses during procedures involving the digestive system. No one knows if it's dangerous to use secretin repeatedly over a long period of time, and no one can truly attest to its safety. This puts at risk the health of many autistic children who are actively seeking this type of treatment. Adverse side effects may take time to appear, and no one knows what to expect.

With these concerns in mind, many doctors and therapists strongly suggest that caution and conservatism prevail when evaluating new regimens. It's acceptable to mix and match therapies, but it's best to rely on ones that are known to be safe and effective. Much of the allure in drugs like secretin is in how relatively easy it is to introduce them into your child's life, rather than the numerous training sessions required for ABA, Floortime, or other similar interventions. It would be wonderful if there was a quick and easy way to help autistic children get better, but in truth, there isn't.

Does it pay to pursue alternative therapies in conjunction with traditional ones?

Because autism is such a complex developmental disorder, and one that affects each child differently, it requires a multi-pronged approach. Accordingly, experts and parents are becoming increasingly more open to non-traditional interventions. But because so many of the complementary therapies are unproved by hard science, they're best paired with the traditional regimens so you can be sure you're covering all the bases.

Know, though, that most alternative therapies have yet to show solid proof that they work. Many of them rely on "success stories" and word-of-mouth, as well as referrals from parents who have witnessed improvements in their children after trying them out. If you're looking to augment your child's educational and therapeutic regimens with alternative programs that will have the same rate of success, you may be disappointed. However, if you're more interested in rounding out your child's schedule so that it includes "fun time" that can stretch his abilities and benefit his mind as well as his body, there's no harm in trying out activities that don't purport to be the "magic bullet" that will cure all of your child's ailments. In a sea of difficulties and therapies, your child should have time simply to be a child and to indulge in a little bit of play, be it in a martial arts studio, on a horse, or on a backyard jungle gym. As long as he has a program in place that addresses the more pressing concerns of autism, his participation in alternative regimens should do no harm. Think of them as enhancements to his life, activities that will bring him joy and expand his horizons.

Before you sign on for any of these therapies (or, for that matter, anything in general), allot some time to do your homework. First, you'll need to assess that the regimen is widely considered safe for children; it's unwise to rely only on what the practitioners or providers tell you. (In an effort to recruit new clients, some providers may not be as forthcoming about matters of safety and efficacy as you might like them to be.) Shop around for the best rates; one martial arts studio may charge astronomical fees, while the same high-quality service and instruction is available elsewhere for less. Beware, too, any claims that insurance will reimburse you for your outlay; each company is different and some are more generous than others. Remember to check with your child's doctor to make sure that the program is appropriate for your child, and that any therapist or staff member who will have direct contact with your child is reputable and has extensive experience caring for children with autism or similar disorders.

ORGANIZING YOUR CHILD'S TREATMENT TEAM

Should we switch to a pediatrician who's more in touch with autism? Or does it not matter because he/she will only treat my child for the usual childhood illnesses?

It can only be advantageous if your child's pediatrician is savvy about autism; this way, you won't have to explain his unusual behaviors at every turn or worry that his doctor may not take his disorder into account when he recommends a procedure or course of treatment. For example, if your child has an ear infection, some physicians may recommend ear drops that will help ease discomfort. Getting medications into the ears of typical children is hard enough; try pinning down an autistic child who doesn't like to be touched or feel enclosed. If your child's doctor isn't familiar with the fears and needs of those with the disorder, he may not understand why you're reluctant to take his advice or even why you're not able to successfully implement his prescription day after day.

A pediatrician who's familiar with autism, on the other hand, will know about your child's quirks; she'll even anticipate that putting drops into your child's ears may only frighten him and that the entire plan will backfire. She knows that, instead of being able to make the patient feel better, the stress of trying to follow her prescribed course of action may make matters only worse. If your child isn't getting the help she needs for her infection, she won't get better. The doctor will have to devise a solution that best fits your child's situation, taking into account that the autism may limit her choices.

That said, it's important to note that it's not easy to find a good doctor. If you're happy with the one you've already chosen for your child, you may find it a challenge to replace someone who's pleasant, attentive, and trustworthy with a healthcare provider in whom you'll have an equal amount of confidence. A doctor who has treated children with the disorder may not necessarily be the best fit for *your* family. Therefore, if you have a physician with whom you've always had a great working relationship, and you'd like to be able to continue consulting her for your children's ailments, consider discussing your concerns with her directly. She may be willing to learn more about autism and thus be able to treat your child much more effectively. Possibly, she may be willing to co-manage your child with whomever you're consulting about autism (a child psychologist perhaps, or a developmental pediatrician), someone who's more familiar with autism and with whom she can share information about your child. Or she may simply be open to your input, and may ask to see any notes or written feedback you've received from the autism experts you're consulting so she's kept apprised of the situation.

If, however, your pediatrician seems uninterested in your child's diagnosis of autism, or if she's been made aware many times of the condition but persists in recommending treatments that clash with your child's sensibilities, it may be time to make the switch. All patients, especially young ones and those who can't quite advocate for themselves, deserve a doctor who listens and cares deeply about their welfare. If a pediatrician doesn't appear to understand how your child's autism impacts his overall health, consider starting over and going elsewhere for routine checkups. Ask the autism expert you've been consulting for recommendations and then interview a few doctors until you find one who knows what the developmental disorder is all about and what it demands.

Aside from developmental pediatricians
   and therapists associated with a specific
   intervention program, who else
   should we be consulting?

Most intervention programs require your child to see a team of experts, which may include a speech therapist, psychologist, psychiatrist, and occupational therapist. If these professionals aren't part of the team, your child's doctor may recommend you consult one or all of them, anyway (your physician will usually offer references, but you can also get names of reputable practitioners from other parents). Here's what you need to know about each of them:

- Speech therapists will work with your child on language development. The strategies recommended will depend largely on the interventions—ABA or Floortime, for example—to which you've subscribed. If the therapist has also diagnosed your child with a condition other than autism that affects his ability to express himself, such as apraxia (in which the mouth can't physically execute the speech signals the brain sends it), the therapist will devise exercises like sucking shakes through a straw to mimic and practice a specific movement of the mouth to address it.
- Psychologists and psychiatrists help identify behavioral and social issues, such as aggression and phobias, that surface due to your child's autism. They can address any emotional difficulties you or your child may be having as you cope with the diagnosis, and may suggest ways that your child can begin to interact more effectively with others. They can also show you how to strengthen family dynamics and manage relationship issues that may arise from caring for a child with autism.
- Occupational therapists help children with autism improve fine and gross motor skills and prescribe regimens that address sensory dysfunctions.

What is the best way to know if a medical or therapeutic provider is right for my autistic child?

You'll know if a doctor or therapist is right for your child if he or she addresses your child's needs and your concerns in a way that's respectful and collaborative. Autism is a diagnosis that affects the entire family and requires it to pull together to find a way to cope; your child's healthcare provider must be aware of this and be able to serve as your guide through the maze of possibilities. Although you may not agree with the doctor's course of action at every turn, it helps if the person is open to dialogue and discussion. Justifiably, you'll have many questions, and they'll need to be taken seriously just as you must seriously place your faith in the doctor's expertise.

Finding the appropriate caregiver will require some work; you may have to interview several candidates before you find one who fits your and your child's style. Take as much time as you need to find the right person, as long as you're not deferring the decision so long that your child suffers from the delay. Ask other parents of autistic children for referrals, and make use of your local special-education district. If your child is already enrolled in one form of intervention, that therapist may be able to make suggestions if you want to investigate someone else for another regimen. It's important to note, however, that no one person may fit the bill completely, especially if you set the bar too high. What's important is that you find someone who's dedicated to helping children with autism, has exhibited a proven track record, and with whose approach you agree.

If, for any reason, you have misgivings about your child's healthcare providers, don't hesitate to voice your concern. A good doctor or therapist should be responsive, provided you approach them in a professional manner. Good communication is key to any relationship, including a doctor-patient one. However, if you feel marginalized or dismissed, something may be amiss. Trust your instincts and start investigating other possibilities; your child deserves the best care possible available.

QUESTIONS TO ASK A POTENTIAL DOCTOR OR THERAPIST

- What experience do you have working with children on the autistic spectrum?
- Do you subscribe to a specific type of intervention—i.e., ABA or Floortime?
- How do you evaluate your patients? What criteria do you use?
- Are you open to alternative approaches?
- How do parents contact you and how quickly do you call them back?
- Do you record your sessions, and if so, can parents get copies for review?
- What is your policy regarding medication?
- What are your hospital affiliations?
- Which insurance plans do you accept?
- Are you certified?
- Do you draw up a personalized therapy plan for each patient, or do you apply a set plan you've established to all of them?
- Do you use a "team approach"? If so, how do you choose the specialists and therapists you work with?
- How often do you re-evaluate my child, and can I get written copies of these reports?
- Are you willing to attend an Individualized Education Plan meeting or, if unable, send a report on my child? (See chapter 8.)
- Are siblings able to participate in the therapies you suggest?
- Do you attend conferences on autism?
- Can you give me a plan to work on at home with my child?
- Do you have any families I can speak to for references?

GAUGING THE SUCCESS OF THERAPY

My child seems to be improving with his
     therapy. Does this mean the worst
     is behind us?

With any luck, it may be. It's difficult to accurately predict the course that
therapy will take. Sometimes improvement is constant and steady, sometimes it may feel like "three steps forward, two steps back." But if your
child is receiving proper and consistent treatment, and his skills are measured and assessed often, it's likely he'll continue to master new skills. He
may reach a point, though, where improvement could plateau for a while,
as some developmental levels are more difficult than others. Adolescence,
for example, and all it entails, may be a challenge for both parent and
child, as it is with many typical teenagers.

Why is my child regressing during a therapy
     that previously has been successful?

Children often regress even as they learn a new skill—it's a trait seen in
children who aren't autistic as well as those who are. Sometimes, in gear-
ing up for a new spurt of development, they appear to take a step back.
But they may just be preparing for the work that the next stage requires.
If you're concerned about your child's progress, check with his doctors
and therapists—they'll have a clearer picture of where he's been and where
he's headed. Sometimes, we want so much for our children to do well that
we're unable to see their entire trajectory, how far they've come, and all
the work they've already accomplished. Participants in his care who are
more objective can help remind us of the victories.

What if, despite all the interventions, my child never gets better?

It's possible, although it doesn't happen often, that in spite of all your efforts, your child sees few gains in the immediate future. It's a painful reality to come to terms with, but some autistic children don't improve, no matter how much intervention or therapy they receive. This scenario, however, is far from the norm, and if you're still in the midst of investigating all the interventions, we urge you to not lose hope. It sometimes takes a little longer than usual to discern the benefits of any regimen. You may have to be more patient. It's normal to feel disheartened after you and your child have made so great an effort, but faith and hope will see you through some of the worst times.

If, however, you and your child have been through a battery of interventions, from educational to medical to alternative regimens, and have yet to see any improvement, discuss this situation with your child's medical and therapeutic team and ask what recourse is left. They may be aware of other avenues you can pursue that haven't yet been made available to you. They may also be able to help you cope with the ongoing disappointment or refer you to a therapist who can help you sort through your emotions. Although you may feel like giving up, consider a short break instead. Perhaps you're exhausted from all the effort, and need time to take care of yourself and renew your energies before you continue the long fight. Try not to lose hope: New interventions are cropping up every day, and in the future you may hit upon a combination that will work wonders for your child.

It helps, too, to manage expectations. Your child may not have made gigantic leaps and bounds developmentally, but he may have made numerous small ones that add up to an impressive whole. Every little bit of progress works toward your overall goal, and if, after all the work, he's able to only make eye contact and nothing else, that's quite an achievement right there. In the deepest, darkest times, celebrate your child and love him the best you can. Although he may still appear unreachable, there's still a chance that you're reaching him on some level, and he's unable to reach back. Love is a powerful force, one that manages to communicate through all sorts of barriers, even autism, and by giving him your all, no matter what measurable results you achieve, he's bound to get better soon, however improvement is defined.

6.

FAMILY AND
RELATIONSHIP ISSUES

. . . .

The dynamics of family life are irrevocably changed once you receive a diagnosis of autism. But this doesn't mean you can't have a fulfilling family and social life. This chapter will help you navigate the tricky maze of relationships while you cope with your child's autistic needs.

How do I explain autism to my child's siblings?

Coming to terms with autism is difficult enough for adults, so you can imagine what a challenge it can be for young children to grasp. That said, kids are amazingly resilient, and if you approach the topic carefully, they'll be able to take the news well. Before you speak with them about their sibling, try to make sense of the diagnosis first yourself. Your other children will look to you for cues about how to respond, and if you appear bereft and inconsolable, they will assume that the future is hopeless and will take that message to heart. But if you present it to them as a challenge to which the family will rise, and express the hope that their autistic sib will receive the help and intervention needed, overcoming most, if not all, the problems that may come your way, then they'll likely feel confident, too. If you don't appear devastated, they have no reason to believe that the diagnosis will be devastating. Instead, they'll adopt your hopeful attitude.

However, it's important to be honest. You don't want to underestimate the challenges that lie ahead; kids need to know what to expect just as adults do. Be as specific as you can but try to convey information with empathy. If you say something that sounds too scary, kids may feel overwhelmed. For example, if they ask, "Did you find out why my sister won't talk to me?" you can reply, "Your sister probably won't be talking anytime soon, but we're seeing specialists who will help her learn how to communicate." That response sounds more positive than "Your sister won't talk to you because she's sick and she can't. I don't know when she will, and she may never say a word—ever."

Make an attempt to keep explanations about the disorder simple. Kris Oudsema, a Belleville, Michigan, mother of three children—one of whom is autistic—explained her son Nick's disorder to her daughters by saying he was "wired differently than other kids so he acts differently. Things that are easy for other kids, like talking and playing, are hard for him." This explanation captures the difficulties of autism succinctly without making them seem insurmountable. Kris and other parents interviewed for this book also emphasized the need to be matter-of-fact about the diagnosis. After all, it's easier for kids to accept someone when it's a given that they should. Children are much more accepting and open to change than we sometimes think they are. Give their kind-heartedness a chance to flourish and it will.

Avoid overwhelming children with details and statistics, as these are likely to confuse them, but leave the door open for questions. They may not ask you questions about the condition immediately, but may do so piecemeal, lobbing you their inquiries as they come up. And if you can't offer any definitive answers, it's okay to say "I don't know."

If it's helpful, and if your autistic child's doctors approve of the idea, bring your other children to some of the appointments. This will take the mystery away and will give them a clearer idea about what you and your autistic child are dealing with when you're not home. During this visit they may also be able to learn how to help; if they're active participants in their sibling's therapies and regimens, they may feel empowered instead of brushed to the side.

However, if any of your children appear deeply upset about the news, prepare yourself to come to their aid. In spite of how much care you take in telling them, they may still find the diagnosis difficult to hear. This may be especially true if your autistic child's disorder is severe. Your other children could feel anger about how their lives have changed since autism entered the family. They may also feel guilty for having negative thoughts and feelings directed toward their autistic sibling. Assure them that their feelings are normal, and that you will all work together to find peace with the diagnosis. Remind them that you're a unit, and that together, you're a force to be reckoned with, even if the foe is autism.

Some books you may want to consult that address the issue are:

- *Autism Through a Sister's Eyes,* by Eve B. Band and Emily Hecht
- *Ian's Walk: A Story about Autism,* by Laurie Lears
- *Andy and His Yellow Frisbee,* by Mary Thompson

How can I make time for all my children when my autistic child's therapies take up so much of my days?

There are only twenty-four hours in a day and, unfortunately, much of that time is occupied by your autistic child's needs. But your other kids need you, too. Short of cloning yourself, you may want to call in the reinforcements. By this we mean taking any and all help you can get from friends, well-meaning relatives, volunteers, organizations that can send aides your way, and anyone you can afford to hire. As much as you'd like to be as hands-on with your autistic child as possible, it's important to be able to delegate some of the work to others who are willing and able. For example, form a carpool with another parent from your autistic child's school so that on some mornings you can breakfast with your other children. Or divide up the appointments with your spouse or partner so that one of you can always attend functions in which your other children are involved, such as recitals or school performances. Have grandma or grandpa host a playdate with your autistic child while you spend time with one of her siblings.

If your household budget permits, hire someone to clean your house or have your laundry professionally done. This frees up a few precious hours for you to devote to your kids so that each gets some quality time from you and your partner. It's great for the entire family to hang out together, but all children, whether they're on the spectrum or not, need some one-on-ones, too. Spend time with them individually so that each of them has your attention without having to compete for it, and encourage them to ask for your time if they feel they need a little more of it. Explain that even though you're not always immediately available, that you'll make time for them in your schedule. As long as they know that they're just as important as your child with autism, your relationship will remain strong and healthy despite the demands of the disorder.

How can I facilitate a good relationship between my autistic and nonautistic children?

"Facilitate" is the right term for your role. Parents with more than one child will tell you that it's what they hope for their children, but a strong and solid relationship has to blossom on its own, under its own steam. Siblings may love each other, but they can't be forced to like each other completely or to be each other's best friend. And when autism enters the picture, the challenge is made that much more complicated. Your other children may feel that the one with ASD receives all the attention, or they may not know how to react to her when she's having difficulties. But there are many things you can do to encourage a healthy bond, one that comes from shared experiences and a genuine understanding of each other's personalities and quirks.

After thoroughly explaining what autism is to your other children, and what they can expect from their sibling, answering any questions they may have about the disorder, help them find ways to become involved in your autistic child's therapies and interventions; this will familiarize them with their sibling's struggles. They'll also feel empowered because they learn how to communicate with their sibling and, consequently, how to read her cues and inspire her to interact with them. Tell them how much you appreciate their efforts, and remind them that although she may not be able to express it, their sibling enjoys and welcomes their presence in her life.

But not everything can be about autism, either. Although it's the focus of your family right now, the needs of your other children must be taken into account as well. If they don't want to participate in an activity or therapy session with your child, then so be it. Let them know that they're always welcome, and that they don't have to join in unless they want to. It's important that they don't feel as if autism always comes first; this way, they won't be overwhelmed by the permanence of the condition.

Respect and appreciate your children as individuals; they are each fashioning their own identities, and crave your approval and support. Avoid comparing them to each other, and celebrate their uniqueness. At the same time, it may be helpful to point out the wonderful characteristics they share, especially if they feel they have nothing in common with their autistic sibling. Remind them of the good times they share with each other, and how there'll be many more as your child with ASD conquers more challenges and gets better over time.

Should we start family therapy to work through the difficulties of caring for an autistic child?

Yes. You and your family are going through a monumentally difficult period in your lives. You're trying to help your autistic child, maintain a relationship with your partner, raise your other children well, and remain sane in the face of troubles and setbacks. Everybody else in your family is carrying a heavy load as well. Plus, the diagnosis has shifted the dynamics of your family; each member is trying to find equilibrium. At a session with a family therapist, everyone gets a chance to air their concerns on neutral ground in front of an objective observer who can help make sense of your emotions. When you try to deal with problems on your own, it's difficult to be objective because you're also deeply involved in the situation. A therapist can identify pockets of trouble and guide each of you toward workable solutions.

In addition to helping steer you through the emotional minefields, a therapist can also help you pay attention to the developments worth celebrating within your family that you're too mired in everyday life to see clearly. He'll be able to illustrate how your family works well together so you can learn from your triumphs and take joy in them. Human nature sometimes makes it difficult to dwell on the good when you're faced with challenges. But with a mental health professional on your family's side, you'll be able to emerge from your experience with autism not only intact, but with strong and improved relationships.

How do I handle negative comments from relatives who think my child is merely "acting out" and don't believe autism is the cause of some of his behavior?

You can approach this problem in several ways. First, assume that their harsh comments stem from a lack of information and by all means make an attempt to correct their misperceptions. Tell them your child has a neurological disorder that makes it hard for your child to respond to sensory stimuli or situations as well as other kids, and that this behavior is neither your child's fault nor yours. Offer to lend them books, pamphlets, and other reading material about autism, or direct them to a few sites on the Web that might clarify their questions. Be evenhanded and matter-of-fact, and try not to let your anger or irritation take over. Although it's not fun to hear your family members blaming your child for something she can't help, they may refrain from doing so again if they come to comprehend what autism is about.

If, however, after numerous attempts they still cannot be more supportive of you and your child, tell them that you may have to refrain from spending time with them if they're unable to keep their negative comments to themselves. Again, your patience and calm are warranted under these circumstances, as anger may only make matters worse. Explain that you won't be avoiding their company simply because you don't like them, but because you find their attitude potentially devastating to your child, who may hear what the relatives are saying or sense their frustrations, and may take their responses to heart. Feel free to share your own pain, as well. Perhaps they don't understand just how hurtful they've been, and may want to work with you toward a resolution.

Nevertheless, if a family member simply cannot find a way to be supportive of you and is continually negative toward your child, then you may need to keep your distance. Prepare yourself for a rocky road, though; severing ties with a family member (or even a friend) isn't easy, and the repercussions may be great. Other relatives may chime in on the feud with their opinions, and feel the need to declare their loyalties. Separating yourself from someone who has refused to lend a hand or make an effort is a last-ditch effort; be sure that you've tried all avenues before you resort to it. If this is where you find yourself, however, take strength in your convictions and know that you're watching out for your child's best interests.

What can my parents do to help out with my autistic child?

Plenty. When it comes to autism, the more people around to celebrate your child, the better. Grandparents can participate in her therapy sessions either at home or in the doctor's office; take your child to the playground or any other places she enjoys for some fun time; or just spend time getting to know her. Most therapists will agree that children, no matter what difficulties they face, thrive on lots of love and attention. Participating in your child's interventions may be helpful for your parents, too; they'll gain hands-on experience and develop skills that will teach them how to interact effectively with your child, which can only help them bond. If you have other children, grandparents can also provide much-needed one-on-one time. They can take each grandchild on "dates," so that everyone gets the attention they deserve.

There are also the more pragmatic considerations. Another pair of hands can be a boon when your schedule is packed with doctors' appointments and therapy sessions, not to mention the usual demands of life. Your parents can take over some of those duties, freeing up some of your time for other responsibilities, or even a little R&R. After all, parents and caregivers of children with ASD need help and support, too. Caring for an autistic child is taxing, no matter how dedicated you are—it drains your emotional reserves and saps your energy. By stepping into your shoes from time to time, your parents can give you some breathing space that allows you to take care of yourself. When you return to your regular duties, you'll be renewed and refreshed. Their assistance can also allow you and your partner some time alone to focus on your relationship, a luxury in families faced with as many demands as yours has.

My marriage has suffered from the challenges of raising an autistic child. How can we get help?

If you feel as if your relationship is crumbling under the weight of the diagnosis and the attendant responsibilities, try investing in some couple time. The pressures placed on a marriage by raising children, especially one with special needs, are great, and couplehood usually suffers. Try not to blame yourself too much, though; unfortunately this happens often. What's important is that you recognize that change needs to happen now.

Keeping the lines of communication open works wonders. Talk to your partner about your concerns about the marriage, and express that you miss spending time with him or her. You'll find that your partner probably feels the same way, and you can then build on your shared emotions. Set aside one night a week or every two weeks when you make time for nothing but each other—hire a sitter, swap babysitting time with other parents, or ask relatives to watch your children while the two of you catch a movie, sit down for a quiet dinner, or go for a walk. If you can, ban all talk of autism and parenting; this is your time to relax and unwind together, not a chance to iron out the logistics of your hectic schedule.

If you feel that your marriage has been damaged and can't be repaired merely by making time for each other, you may need to consult a marriage therapist. Ask your child's doctors and therapists for a referral, and try to find someone with experience working with couples who have faced challenges similar to yours. (If this isn't possible, a reputable marriage counselor should do the trick.) And, remember, there's no shame in facing your discord head-on. To seek counseling is only a testament to your commitment to each other and the welfare of your family. Think of it this way: When your car breaks down, you take it to a mechanic. When your relationship suffers, you take it to a professional who can help you fix the problems before the entire "vehicle" falls apart for good.

My partner and I are getting separated. How do we make this difficult time more manageable for our autistic child?

A family therapist experienced with helping families with special needs would be able to provide the best suggestions on how to navigate this difficult terrain. But here are some points to remember: Separation and divorce are hard on couples, sometimes even harder on their children, autistic or not. And no matter how you approach the issue, it will be a painful process. Your child's reaction will depend on how you both choose to break the news to her, and where she is on the spectrum. If she's high-functioning, she may be able to comprehend your reasons for separating and may even discern that the decision was difficult to make and that you both have her welfare in mind. But if she's severely autistic and barely communicates and doesn't show that she's digesting what you're saying, you may have a harder time trying to gauge how she's processing the news.

Understand, too, that your child may react to the news in ways for which you weren't prepared: Even if she doesn't say anything, she can probably sense that a big change is in the offing, and if she's not able to express her fears and concerns, she may act out her turmoil instead. She may regress in some behaviors, appearing to have lost certain skills she has mastered, or she may withdraw into her world more than usual. On the other hand, she may appear unfazed, only to later react more strongly that you ever imagined.

Handle her with much patience and tenderness. Like any child, she's trying to grapple with adult problems that are overwhelming and perplexing. But unlike other kids, she may not have all the tools she needs to cope with the sadness and complications that have befallen her family. She also needs to know that both her parents will be available to her, no matter what, and that although you may no longer all live under one roof, she can expect much of her routine to stay intact. Autistic children thrive on sameness, and if too much shifts at one time, she may not be able to adjust to the new situation at all.

Can my friendships with parents of children who aren't autistic stay intact?

Most likely, yes, but it may take some work to maintain friendships, especially in the early stages when you've just heard the diagnosis. Autism tests not only your family, it tests your friendships, too. For one thing, you probably won't be as available to your friends as you used to be. Your life will be filled with many commitments, exponentially even more than other parents with typical children have.

Also, expect tension to creep into your relationships as your grief may include moments when you look at your friends' lives and say, "They've got it so much easier than I do, and it's not fair." This is normal; you're stunned by the enormity of the challenges that face your child, and wish you could avoid them if you could. It's understandable that you would feel sad, and being around your friends may remind you of the injustice of it all, and consequently, you'll likely want to avoid them for a while. Acknowledge your emotions and allow them time to settle, but be sure to discuss them with your friends. They won't be able to understand what you're going through unless you explain it to them. After all, good friendships can withstand many storms, but not without open communication. Make an effort not to direct your anger over the diagnosis at your friends—they aren't to blame. On the contrary, you'll need their support to get through this difficult time.

Be prepared, too, for their reactions. Although they love you and your family, they may not know what to say or how to express their grief clearly. They may come at you with suggestions, trying to help, when all they really want to let you know is that they're available to you when you need them. They may also feel some guilt over having children who aren't on the spectrum and not know how to deal with it. They may even worry that they're hurting your feelings by their very presence, prompting them to keep their distance, waiting to take their cue from you. They may fret that their children won't know how to act around your child and may do something wrong. In trying to spare your child's emotions, they may keep their children away from yours, or may watch them like a hawk to make sure they treat your child "correctly," as best they understand what "correctly" means. Their awkwardness may be apparent, and make them appear inconsiderate or uncomfortable.

Keep in mind, though, that if they are good friends, they too will feel saddened by the news. Their sadness may never match yours, but if they care for you then most likely they care a lot for your child too, and knowing that someone important to them has been diagnosed with a serious developmental disorder will probably devastate them as well. Encourage them to talk about their feelings and discuss any concerns they have; offer to educate them about the disorder so that they and their children will know how to relate to your child better. Trust that their intentions are good, unless proven otherwise, and suggest books or Web sites for them to consult for information.

Problems have a way of taking over our lives, and when we're deeply mired in them, it's easy to let them overwhelm us. You can't expect your friend to listen to your toils and troubles all the time without you reciprocating. Although your life may have taken a cruel turn, your problems shouldn't always trump theirs. Sometimes, friendships fall into a certain dynamic wherein the person with the perceived "more serious" problems begins to feel as if nothing else can compare to their suffering. Conversely, the other person grows fatigued from constantly having to give support but being fearful to discuss their own troubles in case they're judged to be bellyaching over comparatively unimportant issues. Competition over "who suffers more" can be damaging in the long run.

The bottom line: healthy friendships are bidirectional, each person taking a turn supporting the other and investing time toward deepening the bond. Not every conversation can be about autism, not every moment shared should dwell on sadness and bad news. If you allow it, your friend can also be your escape, someone who'll encourage you to believe that the world is full of hope and possibilities.

7.

PARENTING AND
LIFESTYLE ISSUES

. . . .

Your child may be autistic, but like all kids, he still needs your guiding hand as he grows up and learns how to get along with others and handle new situations. This chapter provides tips on strategies for the challenges every parent faces, but which poses unique problems for those of an autistic child.

How do I appropriately discipline my child?

Discipline is one arena where the input from your child's medical, therapeutic, and educational support group matters a lot. It's tricky enough to figure out how to discipline any child, let alone one who is grappling with numerous speech and sensory issues. Your child's teachers and healthcare providers will be able to provide suggestions tailor-made for your child's abilities and needs.

One strategy that has worked for families involves the use of a designated chair in which a child is asked to sit for a certain amount of "quiet time." A clock or a timer left in plain view of the child, one that shows how much time is passing, helps a child know how long he must remain seated and helps divert him for the duration. If he can be left alone in a chair in a quiet room where he can't hurt himself, this method may work well.

But for some children with ASD, this approach will backfire. Instead of sitting quietly, a child may become even more worked up and trash the room they're in. Some parents use a "deep pressure response," in which they hold their child or even sit on them (not out of anger and with complete awareness of how much pressure they're applying) to give a child the sensory input needed to calm down. Before you embark on this type of approach, check with your child's pediatrician on how it should best be implemented. It's not meant as punishment, but as a way to soothe kids with underdeveloped tactile senses.

If your child is high-functioning, you may be able to rely on a reward system by which a favorite object is taken away when he acts out, but is given back when he corrects his behavior.

With the help of experts, you'll be able to devise a disciplinary approach that works well for your child. One thing's clear, however: Corporal punishment (that is, hitting or spanking), which already is a sensitive parenting subject that has stirred much debate, probably has no place in a home where a child on the spectrum is present. Your child will most likely be unable to comprehend why he's being spanked, and may see it only as aggressive behavior on your part, inciting fear and mistrust in him. Besides, if he's sensitive to touch, a light spanking may feel like a beating to him, and he may believe he's under siege, triggering the very responses you're trying to stop (biting, kicking, or screaming, for example). It's important to be patient; autism is a developmental disorder that affects communication and interaction, and discipline is such a complex concept that he's bound to have difficulty understanding what you're trying to teach him.

Is it reasonable for me to set rules for my autistic child?

Yes, as long as they take into account your child's developmental level. Your child needs limits and boundaries just like any other, perhaps even more so if he's unable to gauge on his own what's safe and what's not. While it may seem easier to follow his lead in everything, he needs you to set standards for him. Be sure to explain your rules clearly. Approach this as a teaching opportunity, a chance to expand his horizons and challenge his skills. And keep the regulations to a minimum—if you give him too many directives, he may become overwhelmed by all of them and follow none. Expect to have to remind him about the rules often; learning how to follow rules is just like any other skill he's trying to acquire, and it may take time for him to get it down. Carol Gray's social stories, which help you find a way to communicate complicated concepts and teach behaviors (see chapter 5 for more information), may work well in this kind of situation, or ask your child's pediatrician for any suggestions.

Once your child understands what you expect from him, remember to give him kudos when he remembers to follow the rules. Consistent reinforcement works wonders in encouraging positive behaviors. Also, you need to abide by your own policies as well; if you appear to waffle on any of them, he may get the idea that rules aren't really important, and won't stick to them. Serve as a model and show him what's appropriate and what's not, and be prepared to adjust the standards if they seem too rigid.

Should I give my child chores (room clean-up, trash duty, etc.) as I would to a nonautistic child?

Definitely, if he can perform them. But know that he may not be able to accomplish as much as you expect, especially if he's moderately or severely autistic. Instead of presenting them as chores, try portraying them as fun activities. If you're making the bed, for example, have him "race" to see how fast he can put the pillows where they belong or let him clean his tub after bath with a washcloth. Celebrate his endeavors and let him know that he's doing a good job, even if it may not be perfect.

Is toilet training more difficult with autistic children?

It's likely that you'll find toilet training more difficult for your child than parents whose kids aren't on the spectrum. Because autistic children do suffer from sensory dysfunction, getting them ready to use the potty, especially for bowel movements, can be a daunting task. Kids may also have motor problems that could make it hard for them to get comfortable on a potty seat or the toilet, adding to the difficulties. However, most children on the spectrum do get toilet-trained, albeit a little later than most typically developing kids. The key is waiting for them to be developmentally ready for the next step, instead of imposing the challenge on them at a predetermined age. Kids without autism are usually ready for toilet-training around the age of two or three, but you may have to wait until your child is five or six (or even older) before he can even comprehend what it means to use the bathroom when he needs to instead of letting it happen spontaneously. Check with your child's developmental pediatrician or psychologist about how to approach toilet training. Strategies will depend on which intervention plan you subscribe to. For more tips, check out *Toilet Training for Individuals with Autism and Related Disorders* by Maria Wheeler.

One way to get children excited about the prospect of toilet training is through books, especially ones that have simple illustrations that can explain what the process entails. Some children's books to try include *Once Upon a Potty* by Alona Frankel (there's one for boys and another for girls) and *The Potty Book* by Alyssa Satin Capucilli. (If your child is older and likes to read, he may want to peruse Mary Wrobel's book, *Taking Care of Myself: A Hygiene, Puberty and Personal Curriculum for Young People with Autism*.) It also helps if he sees you or your partner model the behavior. Be prepared to answer questions as he may find the process both confusing and fascinating.

Q. Do we need to take special precautions when childproofing our home for our autistic child?

Whether or not you have an autistic child, you should always follow the basic rules of safety and childproof your home from top to bottom. In addition, there are special precautions you may have to take because your child's on the spectrum. For one, many ASD kids have been to known to "escape" rooms and homes when they're under stress from people or sensory input they can't manage to process. Consider installing a dead bolt out of your child's reach on the front and back doors to prevent him from wandering out on his own, or alarm systems that will alert you if he's managed to work the locks and leave your home.

If your child seems unusually attracted to objects that can be dangerous and that are usually found in one area, such as knives in the kitchen, hide them from him so he won't be able to hurt himself. Autistic kids often have sensory issues that prevent them from realizing something is a danger, like not being able to feel pain as strongly as they normally would. For these kids, placing a hand on a stovetop that has been left on, for example, won't necessarily teach them to move their hand away before it burns, so you will need to observe them closely and use your judgment to determine what may cause a problem later.

How do I teach my child about safety issues like strangers and bullies?

There are many ways to alert your child to the dangers of strangers and bullies. You can use social stories (see chapter 5), drawings to teach them to handle situations that can be purchased or that you can make yourself that show cause and effect in a given situation. You can also model behavior through action figures and toys. But the best way to inform your child about safety is to work with your child's therapist and teachers to reinforce the message that some people he or she encounters may not have the youngster's best interests in mind. It's a complex concept to teach typical children, and due to communication obstacles you will have unique challenges when discussing safety with your child. You'll have an easier time helping him navigate this minefield if you enlist the help of as many members of his support system as you can.

How do I arrange playdates?

Arranging playdates is fairly simple. If you meet a child with whom yours has taken an interest, no matter how slight, go for it. Your child will benefit from the socializing, might possibly forge a lifelong friendship, and at the very least, he'll have some fun. It's best, however, to keep the playdate group small, as autistic children tend to feel overwhelmed quickly by being around too many people. Having two or three children hang out together is an optimum number, at least to start.

A good playdate, whether the children are autistic or not, requires some structure and clear expectations but allows for exploration and creativity. In order to avoid pitfalls, it helps if you know what the kids will be doing to occupy themselves and how their personalities mesh. This way, you can select activities that both of them like, and thus avoid skirmishes later on, such as having to share toys or agreeing on a group activity. You may want to put away any playthings you know your child will absolutely not tolerate sharing, and have a handful of choices so they don't fight over the one or two toys available.

Although many children on the spectrum are nonverbal and will probably play side by side rather than with each other or engage in imaginative play, it'll help if you set up "play stations" in different areas so they can find an activity they enjoy. Be on the lookout for behaviors such as hand-flapping or spinning that signal that your child has had enough, and head off these occasions at the pass when you can, to avoid major blowouts.

If your child has been invited to a friend's home, bring favorite items that give comfort—a stuffed animal perhaps, or a favorite book. Set guidelines and communicate them to him clearly—for example, say "no outdoors" if you have a little escape artist. Inform your host of the possible pitfalls: Explain that windows and doors will need to be locked, for example, or that certain sights, sounds, or smells are upsetting to your child. Point out to friends and typically developing children how much your child will learn from them and how much they will learn from you and your child.

How do I prepare my autistic child for the hoopla of holidays?

Holidays, although lots of fun, can be tough, even for children who aren't autistic. Days are hectic and packed with errands and appointments, and everywhere you go, it seems that people are rushing about trying to prepare for Christmas, Hanukkah, or Kwanzaa. Lights are everywhere, music filters through nearly every public space, and everyone—grown-ups and little ones—are pumped up. No wonder, then, that many children with ASD find this period especially challenging. They're excited by the commotion, but are likely to be overstimulated, too, especially if they're struggling with sensory integration issues.

While there's certainly no need to avoid being festive altogether, it's important to be aware of your child's needs during this special time. If you must be in the thick of things because of your obligations—shopping, parties, and other functions—be sure your child has a few hours in his day to be at home, where he feels most safe and doesn't have to deal with much activity. Keep his environment serene and allow him to choose what he wants to do during his down time. It's all too easy to let the rush sweep you away but, like everybody else, your child needs to be able to find some peace amid the bustle so he can recharge and conserve his energies. Also, choose carefully which events he truly must attend; much as it would be fun to accept every single invitation that comes your way, socializing is extremely exhausting, autism or no autism. Being present at each and every event will sap your reserves and make your child more apt to act out. Take the holidays day by day, and try to minimize unnecessary chaos. He'll be able to enjoy all the hoopla if he's relaxed and fully rested, not when he's stretched to the limit.

If an obligation is unavoidable and you're visiting someone else's home, and you anticipate that your child may display some behaviors your hosts may not understand, warn them ahead of time about what to expect. Remind them that the holidays can be stressful, and that if your child appears to have had enough of being around groups of people, you may want to seek refuge in a quiet room in another corner of the house, or may leave altogether. When hosts know to anticipate your child's reactions, they're less likely to take offense if you make unusual requests or remove yourself from the celebrations. They'll know what's behind your actions and may just turn out to be more accommodating than you expected.

You may also want to bring your child's favorite foods to holiday events, in case there's nothing made available that he would like to eat. Being in the middle of a raucous party isn't the place to test your child's ability to try new foods; the more comfortable he's made to feel, the more successful your holiday outings will be.

Can my child ever be left with a babysitter?

Yes, as long as it's someone whom you trust and who completely understands what's expected of her as a caregiver for an autistic youngster. Before you hire anybody, make certain you've screened him or her properly and adequately; you can't be too careful with your children, especially if yours is a nonverbal autistic child who cannot easily relay to you any issues that may have arisen when you were not around.

Once you've done the appropriate background and reference checks and have picked someone to help you care for your child, provide her with reading materials about autism and take her with you to your next appointment with the pediatrician. Even if she has some experience with autistic kids, she needs to know how *your* family approaches *your* child's treatment. The children she has previously worked with may have relied on different regimens that required different responses to behavioral issues that came up. Train her in your family's methods of teaching your child so she develops her own expertise. Encourage her to ask questions and let her know of your child's "hot spots," things or events that may upset or anger him.

If your child hasn't met her yet, invite her to spend some time (paid, of course) playing with your child while you're around. This will help your child build trust and give you an idea of what the sitter will be like. Offer constructive criticism when necessary, and compliment her when she does something that works well. Your feedback will be crucial to her success as your child's babysitter.

When you're ready to leave her alone, be sure to let your child know when you're going and how long you'll be away. Sneaking off when he isn't looking will only upset him; it's too abrupt a transition. Let him know that he's with someone he likes and you trust, and appear positive and encouraging. If you're tearful and apprehensive during good-byes, he may feel as if there's something wrong and the session may not go well. Before you leave, set up plenty of activities to occupy him, and be sure to give your babysitter clear instructions on how and where to contact you in case you're needed.

What's the easiest way for me to let others know my child has autism without having to go into the details of the disorder?

Sign up for free with the National Autism Registry (NARY) and ask for business cards that you can flash to people who may not know of, or understand, autism but seem concerned about your child. A sample statement, written by a NARY therapist, Valerie Herskowitz, reads: "This child has autism. Autistic individuals may experience difficulty in certain situations that may cause them to exhibit undesirable behaviors. These outbursts often happen for no apparent reason, or may be due to the individual's inability to tolerate the present environment. The occurrence of these tantrums is a symptom of this syndrome and not due to a lack of appropriate parenting skills."

If you don't have the cards, you can also write a short statement yourself and print them out on fliers that you can distribute; or, when asked, you might say, "My child has a neurological disorder called autism, and he's having a hard time right now. Thanks for your concern." Although this statement usually works in most cases, some strangers, surprisingly, may push for more information. If this is the case and they seem genuinely interested in learning more, spend a little time discussing the disorder with them if you're inclined. If their questions become rude or intrusive, feel free to cut the conversation short and move on. You don't have to explain your child's behaviors if you don't feel like it. Just as other parents aren't under any obligation to apologize for or discuss their kids' meltdowns and tantrums, neither are you and your partner.

How do I get my child to wear a seat belt?

It takes months of patience and practice, but this is one habit that your child must keep. Seat belts aren't only required by law, they also keep him safe. If he's extremely agitated when you buckle him in, try to distract him so he can focus on something else. Tell him a story or hand him his favorite toy, preferably something he can play with right then and there, such as a deck of cards, a handheld game, or a puzzle. Make a big show of buckling his favorite stuffed animal right next to him, or of fastening your own belt. Sometimes, the culprit may not be the seat belt itself, but the general atmosphere in the car. Other passengers may be speaking too loudly, or the volume of the radio may be too high. The windshield wipers may be going too fast, or the wind whistling through the crack in the window may feel too piercing. Experiment to nail down exactly what's bothering him, and respond accordingly. A reward system may also work; show him how you add a sticker to the reward board at home and let him know that when he gets five (or ten, or whatever number you choose), he receives a special treat, such as an ice cream cone or a new toy car.

How do I help my autistic child handle a long plane, train, bus, or car ride?

It's hard to feel like you're having fun when you're sitting down for hours, sometimes strapped in a seat belt, whether it's in a car, bus, plane, or train. But there are some things you can do to make getting to your destination more palatable for your child. First, be sure to pack all his favorite toys, books, foods, and other comfort items and have them within easy reach. If he's kept busy and his attention is diverted during the journey, you're bound to encounter fewer problems than if he's bored and restless. Portable DVDs and handheld games can be pricey, but if you can make the investment and your child enjoys watching movies or playing games, they may be worthwhile.

If you're taking the car, schedule frequent stops along the route for bathroom trips and time to stretch and blow off steam. Perhaps you could chart a course that includes interesting sights that your child may enjoy; even a local playground will help break up the boredom of a long car ride

and give your child some much-needed fun time. Buses are more challenging as they're apt to be crowded and can be uncomfortable, but pack-
ing an arsenal of fun stuff should help. (If you can avoid them, you may
want to avoid buses, unless your child seems to especially enjoy this mode
of transportation.)

Airplanes, although a lot more comfortable, can be challenging. Air-
port security checks require long waits but if you remember to flash your
NARY card stating your child is autistic, you may be able to get to the
front of the line. Onboard, however, your child may have to remain seated
and buckled in for most of the trip, and takeoff and landing may trigger
pain in his ears, which could bring on a meltdown. Trains are easier, as you
can walk around and satiate hunger and thirst in the dining car. Your child
may also find the movement of the train soothing.

How can I tell if my child's feeling overwhelmed and about to melt down in public?

You'll know when your child is having a hard time—his hands may start
flapping, he may grow more active or restless, or he may begin to display
behaviors you've long associated with tantrums. Anticipate the possibility
of a big meltdown by paying close attention to his cues, especially if you're
someplace chaotic or hectic. He'll start letting you know as soon as possible that the outing isn't sitting well with him. His signal may be something
as small as the shaking of a leg or making less eye contact than usual. He
may be more silent or rowdy, or appear confused and listless. If he's verbal
and he says he wants to leave or do something you've associated with his
need to seek comfort, heed his call immediately. When an autistic child says
he doesn't want to participate in an activity anymore—for example, you're
at a birthday party and he says he won't sing and wants everyone to stop
belting out "happy birthday"—it's time to gently whisk him away and let
him find solace elsewhere. He means what he says and it's important that
you listen.

Which places may trigger difficulties for my autistic child?

Most individuals on the spectrum can't abide crowded and noisy venues (unless, of course, your destination is related to a passion of his, such as a baseball stadium if he is a fan of the game). Steer clear of such places if possible, or try to stake out a spot where you're somewhat removed from the fray. In general, though, there are no hard-and-fast rules. Some children, for example, may enjoy swimming; others, however, can't be coerced to go anywhere near a pool or open water. Others may enjoy car rides, whereas some kids consider their car seats the ultimate torture machines. Your child has his own unique set of preferences and dislikes, and you know best what he'll be comfortable with and what will upset him. Follow his lead and in time you'll learn which destinations will be enjoyable and which ones to avoid completely.

What is the Americans with Disabilities Act and how can it help my child?

The Americans with Disabilities Act (ADA), a law enacted in 1990, protects your child's rights, as well as those of other citizens with special needs. It ensures that your child and others like him have unfettered access, as others do, to services provided to the general public. They can't be prevented from seeking housing, using transportation, applying for and acquiring jobs, enrolling in schools, visiting and patronizing commercial businesses, or from participating in most activities sanctioned by state and local entities. It also means that reasonable accommodations should be made for your child. For example, you can't be thrown out of restaurants if your child is having a meltdown and the owners don't understand (or even care about) the nature of autism, and you shouldn't be made to feel unwelcome in public venues. If a place of business doesn't comply, they're subject to fines and other penalties as outlined by the ADA. For more information, contact the ADA information line at the United States Department of Justice at 800-514-0301 / 800-514-0383 (TTY), or visit their Web site at www.ada.gov.

PROTECTING YOUR CHILD'S RIGHTS

· · · · ·

If you feel that your child's rights as outlined in the Americans with Disabilities Act have been violated, you can contact one of the nine federal agencies designated by the ADA to investigate disability-related discrimination complaints filed against state and local government programs. These agencies look into claims of noncompliance related to the following: agriculture; education; employment; health and human services; housing; labor and workforce participation; lands, resources, and environment; transportation; other government functions. They also investigate complaints involving the programs they fund. To obtain contact information for each agency, visit the ADA Web site: www.ada.gov/investag.htm.

8.

YOUR CHILD'S
EDUCATION

. . . .

You are your child's best advocate as he wends his way through the educational system. Find out how you can work with state and local governments, administrators, therapists, and teachers to ensure that he gets the academic support he needs as early as his preschool years.

How are my child's educational rights protected?

Thanks to the Individuals with Disabilities Education Act (IDEA), a law passed in 1975 and heavily amended in 1997, children with special needs (including autistic kids, who are specifically mentioned) age three and above have a right to a "free and appropriate" education. Funded by the government, these special education programs are supposed to meet certain standards set by the Department of Education, should be available at no cost to the parents (usually via the public schools), and should address children's educational needs, including having to provide services that help them learn (such as occupational or speech therapy). As can be expected, "appropriate" means different things to different people, and figuring out what's appropriate for your child depends on three things: your opinion, an assessment made by special-education teachers and administrators from your local schools, and input from therapists and healthcare providers. You'll need to cooperate with a team of experts to devise a plan that you feel will work best for your child.

IDEA also mandates that education occur in the "least restrictive environment." This means that your child should be able to interact with typically developing children as much as possible, and not be segregated from them. Special-education children should be able to learn the same subjects as typically developing kids, and have access to the tools and supports needed for them to succeed in school. While this part of the law helps ensure that children who are handicapped by a disability or disorder are treated equally, it also encourages mainstreaming, which may work for most autistic kids but not for a select few.

How do I know if a school is the right one for my child?

There's no way to make a sound decision about your child's education unless you visit schools, interview teachers, and talk to the parents who have enrolled their kids there. This step is important because brochures, Web sites, or phone calls can't tell you whether a place will nurture your child and provide her with the help and guidance she needs. All good schools should provide a tour for parents, and include a question-and-answer session for them during which administrators and teachers field and respond to questions. When you tour a prospective school, bring with you the list of questions provided in the inset on page 123 and be sure to take notes while you're there.

Also, take time to observe how teachers and staff members interact with the students. Are they approachable but firm? Helpful but not overbearing? Kind and courteous? These are some of the basic hallmarks of a good school. Observe whether or not kids seem happy at the school. It's very telling if the students don't appear to enjoy their activities. Get a feel for the typical class size, and remember that the smaller the better, because that way kids get more attention. Ask how teachers and administrators handle kids who are acting out. Any whiff of corporal punishment is a no-no. And last, but certainly not the least, keep in mind that a place that values your contributions will probably work best in the long run, so try to find a school that encourages parent involvement. If possible, arrange for your child to visit the school as well. You can glean a lot from observing how your child fits into a place and how the teachers and children respond to him.

QUESTIONS TO ASK SCHOOL ADMINISTRATORS TO EVALUATE YOUR CHILD'S POTENTIAL SCHOOL

. . . . .

- What is the teacher-to-child ratio?
- What special education programs are available?
- How is the curriculum set and how does it compare to regular classrooms in the same grade?
- What is the success rate of children in the program moving to an inclusive setting?
- Do the kids have access to the same resources and extracurricular programs as "regular" students?
- How often do children socialize with students in regular classes and how is that facilitated?
- What's the protocol if my child's having an emotional day?
- How do you handle kids who act out?
- How open are you to suggestions from parents?
- Are parents allowed to drop by for a visit, and if so, how often?

Ask to be referred to parents of some of the students, and if you can, approach a parent during drop-off or pick-up and request their candid estimation of the school. Administrators will, understandably, speak highly of the place where they work, but other moms and dads will likely be more willing to give you their honest opinion, especially when no staff members are around.

Trust your instincts. If a school seems great on paper and stellar during a visit, but just hasn't wowed you, go with your gut. Some of the deal-makers we look for can't be quantified. It may come down to the fact that you at once felt comfortable when you visited the school, and knew without a doubt it was the place for your child.

Will my child get the same education as kids who are in a mainstream classroom?

Autistic children may not get the same exact curriculum as children in typical classrooms, but their curriculum will have to meet the standards set by the state for particular grade levels and for special-education students. They won't be allowed to attend a program in which they won't learn anything, which should come as a relief to many parents who worry that their children will fall through the proverbial cracks in the system.

The teaching approach will also be slightly different, addressing problem areas specific to the population. In a classroom designed to serve children on the spectrum, ideally, there will be more tools that address the sensory needs of students, especially as this is an area in which many students display a deficit. Teachers will be trained in ways that elicit communication, the Achilles heel of many ASD kids.

Is my local school district mandated to provide my child with a good education?

"Good" is a relative term. Your school district considers it a top priority to provide the area's children with the best education. In truth, it's only required to provide your child with schooling that meets certain minimum standards, not necessarily the best. Quality can vary from district to district, from state to state. Unfortunately, you have to investigate by calling other parents with children enrolled in the district or scheduling tours to gauge whether your local schools are up to par, a responsibility that parents of typically developing children also have to take on. But trust that you and the rest of the educational team for your child have the child's best interests in mind. If you truly feel your child will be under-served, refuse to settle for anything less than what you think a sound education requires. For more about how to work with your child's educational team, see "What is an IEP?" on page 127.

Does my child need to continue appointments with speech therapists and other clinicians if she's enrolled in a good public school program?

Probably. Even if you find a program within your public school system that serves the needs of your child, it's important to remember that the service won't be able to match a private treatment center where all her needs are met. Public schools can't provide as many one-on-one hours with a clinician as a child who is accustomed to private treatment may be used to. After all, public school systems, no matter how highly rated, have budgets to maintain that constrain "extras" such as speech and occupational therapy. And if your child's written education plan (see "What is an IEP?" on page 127) doesn't indicate that these services are absolutely required—which means they may not be provided for free by the school district—you may have to seek them out on your own. If you're able to afford them, supplementary therapies, if warranted, can only help your child continue to learn and grow.

Will my child receive the same quality education in a special-education classroom as that found in mainstream classrooms?

Ideally, yes. And in some cases, she may get an education of even better quality. Many experts say this is especially true during the preschool years, and children who are on the spectrum are usually referred to schools that are specifically knowledgeable at teaching ASD kids. Teachers in such schools are more likely to be savvy about the issues facing children with the disorder, and can better help them master specific skills and make developmental leaps.

During the elementary years (and older), the challenge to provide a top-rate education is enormous, and the obstacles are equally great, especially for public schools. Districts are faced with shrinking budgets not just for special education but general programs as well, and can't always provide everything a child needs to be successful at whatever cost. And yet, many public schools are able to do what sometimes seems impossible—provide children with special needs the same stellar approach that they employ in all the other schools in their district.

On the flip side, unfortunately, many school districts are struggling to meet the needs of their entire student population, let alone those with special needs. The programs they offer may meet the minimum standards, but fail to rise above them. And if that is what's available to you and your family, you should rightfully consider other options—perhaps a private school that, one hopes, will be paid for by the district. (Or, if you can afford it, one whose financial demands you'll assume yourself.) At the very least, you should attempt to negotiate that the school district provide many ancillary services that supplement what your child may be missing from the school's special-education program.

The bottom line: It's imperative that your child receive a proper, quality education that's appropriate for her. And it's your right to seek out those educational opportunities. With some research and hard work investigating all the options—public or private—you'll be able to come up with a solution that will work well for your family.

What is an IEP?

IEP stands for the "Individualized Education Plan," which is essentially a detailed document that fully specifies the strategy for your child's schooling. A necessary component in receiving special education from your local schools, it outlines not only which classes he'll be taking and in what setting, but establishes his current abilities (what he's capable of doing academically at the time the IEP is written), sets academic goals, and lists the measures by which he'll be evaluated. It also states the dates covered by the plan (which may be a school year), specifies which additional services will be provided (including speech and occupational therapy), and includes any comments you or your partner (or any other relatives directly involved in your child's care) may want to put into the record.

Everyone involved in the education of your child participates in the formulation of the IEP, including teachers and school officials. It may take just one meeting to come up with a document that hits all the marks, or the process may take days; it's as complicated as any contract, because that's what the IEP is—a legal document that addresses all of your child's educational needs. What's mentioned in the IEP is what is carried out, at least until such time as it's necessary to re-evaluate and revise. If you've never been to an IEP meeting before, you may find the minutiae overwhelming. Nearly every single aspect of your child's instruction will be spelled out, down to how many hours of learning he'll be receiving or any equipment a teacher may need to make the classroom experience more productive. (For example, if he's hearing impaired in addition to also being labeled autistic, the IEP may mention a teacher's use of an FM amplification microphone system to talk to him, so he can better make out what she's explaining.) It's a daunting task, even for those who've been through it already. But it makes sense to be precise because what is written down is what your child gets—ambiguity can only lead to future problems.

The writing of an IEP can be as contentious as most contract negotiations, too; sometimes parents may envision one type of strategy and school administrators may picture another. For example, you may be seeking an IEP that states that your child may also receive ancillary services, such as one-on-one tutoring and special sessions for behavioral interventions that you deem important for your child to succeed at school. The school district's representatives, on the other hand, may think an integrated classroom setting fits the bill, and decide that they don't have to pull your child aside for any additional services. In this case, prepare for lots of push-and-pull. Any extras you may request, and which the school district agrees to provide, will have to be funded—at least partially—by the schools themselves.

Your conflicting suggestions may also fly in the face of what school officials have already put in place within the district. After evaluating the programs presently available at their public schools, some parents may find them lacking, which in turn spurs them to find alternative private educational settings, for which tuition they request the public school system pay. In these types of situations, cost will certainly be an issue, and you will discover that there is a fundamental difference in philosophies between you and the school district. Administrators may feel that they have a fine special-education program in place, while what you're indicating by your demands is that it's unacceptable for your child.

When faced with a battle over the IEP, remember that if you have done the proper research and legwork, you are just as qualified as educators to discern what's best for your child and to have a full and sound education paid for by the government. You have a right to make changes prior to signing off on the IEP's final wording and to suggest other programs and assistance. You may not get everything you ask for, but it's certainly worth the fight, especially if you truly feel that accepting what the local schools have to offer may adversely affect your child's mental, physical, and emotional development.

As with nearly every other service your autistic child needs, you need to be his best advocate. To do the job well, you'll need to be armed with all sorts of documentation to back up your requirements. Have handy any letters and records supporting your position from physicians, therapists, psychologists, as well as anyone else on your child's medical team who is familiar with his strengths and weaknesses. If necessary, bring a lawyer to the meetings who will represent your family's interests (we strongly suggest this in extreme cases when an all-out war appears to be inevitable).

However, it's just as important to consider that teachers and administrators are also experts in the field, especially if they specialize in educating children with special needs, autism in particular. They have seen what their programs can do, and know how many other students they've served well. If your child has been in the school system previously, they're aware of his abilities. And remember that they do have your child's interest in mind, at the very least by letter of the law. They're required to make sure their approach is customized for your child, not something generic they foist on all autistic kids who go through the system.

What is an IFSP?

An Individualized Family Service Plan (IFSP) is very similar to an IEP, except that it's drawn up for children from birth to age three who are identified as having special needs. Parents and social service providers work together to write up the document, which specifies what interventions a baby or toddler will receive to address the diagnosis, and makes certain that such services occur in the child's "natural environment"—usually the home—as much as is feasible.

Because the focus of an IFSP isn't mainly on academic learning from preschool onward, it also takes into account what a child's family members need for them to be able to support and help their disabled child learn and grow. In addition to detailing which services a child needs in order to take on developmental challenges and work toward mastering them, it may also include provisions for family therapy, counseling for siblings who may need help coping with the diagnosis, training for all family members in the proper care of children with special needs, and more. As the family adjusts to the situation and the child begins to benefit from interventions, the IFSP is amended, usually every six months.

Is homeschooling a viable alternative for my autistic child?

In some instances, yes, but much depends on your child's abilities and skills. If your child is severely autistic and will benefit most from one-on-one sessions at home, at least initially, then homeschooling may be your best bet. But other experts say that for most children on the spectrum who have been diagnosed as moderate or high-functioning, homeschooling may be a disservice. Their reasoning stems from the belief that children who are autistic and who don't display significant cognitive delays, but have lots of trouble in the social arena, will be able to spend the bulk of their time at a school. There they can develop skills they badly need, and will begin to enjoy interacting with others. Were you to keep them at home most of the time, they wouldn't be able to practice socializing with their peers, and could suffer from the isolation.

In many ways, however, homeschooling can be a godsend. If after much investigation you find that your local school district's special education opportunities are wanting, this may be a great option for you. If you truly feel that the classrooms, teachers, or lesson plans are inadequate or inappropriate for your child, it's understandable that you'd want to consider taking charge of your child's education instead of entrusting it to a public school. Parents have also opted for homeschooling when they don't believe that the philosophy behind a public school program or the interventions offered are right for their child. Similarly if parents' attempts to get the public school to foot the cost of private school tuition are rejected, and they are unable to pay for tuition out of pocket, homeschooling may be the best solution.

If you decide to go this route, take great care to include enrichment activities in your child's schedule, to give her plenty of opportunity to meet and interact with kids her age. It's important that her social needs are met, and that she's able to challenge herself not only academically but emotionally. Many of the challenges faced by children on the spectrum concern their ability to communicate and interact with others; giving them the opportunity to improve in these areas can do wonders for their development.

For more information on this subject, visit www.home-school.com.

My child's teachers say she's ready for a mainstream classroom. Will this be good for her?

We understand your concern: If you've been blessed with a successful IEP that included numerous one-on-one sessions that addressed much of your child's learning deficiencies, you may be reluctant to tinker with a proven formula. You may worry that your child could get lost in the mainstream classroom shuffle, where the child-to-teacher ratios aren't as small as her old classroom and she'll have to deal with kids who may not react kindly to autism. You may be concerned that the teachers, who aren't trained specifically in special education, may not be adequately equipped to guide children with special needs through the lessons and activities.

All of your worries make sense, but try to be receptive to your IEP team's suggestions. They have numerous years of experience in education, and their recommendations are based on what is hopefully an accurate assessment of your child's goals and achievements. Besides, change can be good; if your child's teachers and therapists have assessed her skills and capabilities and recommended that she face the new challenge of being in a mainstream classroom, it likely means that she's progressing well and they think she's ready for an environment in which she spends more hours with her typically developing peers.

How do I plan for my child's educational future after high school?

Unfortunately, once your child graduates from high school, the options for her education may be more limited than you've been used to thus far. Much depends on your child's developmental abilities. If, for example, she's been part of a mainstream classroom for years and has done well with her studies, she may be able to attend a community college or university for a higher degree. She may have to live at home and commute, or, if she's able, room with other teens in dormitories and apartments. Much hinges on the strides she's made through the years. If she's fairly high functioning, she can go as far as she's willing and you needn't believe that there is an end point to her aspirations. The sky's the limit, in a way, if she's been able to find a way to live with disorder.

On the other hand, if your child still needs considerable help by the time she turns eighteen and is done with her K–12 education, or has been unable to earn a high school diploma, you may have to consider another path entirely. Some programs for autistic adults train them for vocational work so they can participate in the workforce. Contact the local chapter of the Autism Society of America for more information on these programs. Many of them are funded by the government; you may not have to pay exorbitant amounts for the training.

Another choice is to find a residential program that can help your child make the transition into adulthood. Such programs include services that will assist in her continued growth and development, and may help her become more independent of you. Unfortunately, some of these businesses have been plagued by complaints about ill-trained staff and poor living conditions, so you will have to do an enormous amount of research to find one you deem suitable. They can also be quite expensive and may not be covered by federal funds or insurance. Check with your state's education department to obtain more information and to determine a program's reputation.

It's never too early to start planning for your child's future. With luck, she'll be able to spread her wings and soar as high as she can because the interventions she's receiving now will help her overcome many of the challenges she is to face in the years ahead. However, it pays to prepare yourself for the eventuality that she may need more assistance as an adult than you'd wished. It is the entire autism community's hope, though, that in ten or twenty years' time, more opportunities will exist for all children on the spectrum, and that many, if not all, of them will have productive, fruitful, and happy lives. In the meantime, you can make a difference by advocating now for that kind of future; volunteer with your local ASA chapter, or with organizations that help children with ASD and their families. By investing in your child's future, you may be able to influence her standard of living in the years to come.

9.

YOUR WORRIES ABOUT
YOUR CHILD'S FUTURE

. . . .

Unfortunately, some of the biggest questions about living with autism are the trickiest. Your anxieties will morph into more complicated ones as your child grows up, but answers lie just around the bend. Here we tackle the most critical concerns about your child's future.

Will my child ever have a best friend?

Quite possibly, yes. Sometimes, it's difficult to imagine that your child, who at times seems barely to be able to connect with you, will find companionship and friendship in someone else. But all signs point to yes, as long as your child is firmly ensconced in therapeutic and educational programs that aim to help him learn how to interact with others and widen his once-tight circle of confidants. In the beginning, he may have been the only one allowed in that circle, but over time and with the proper tools, the boundaries of that small area tend to widen and the circle grows. Soon, he'll be able not only to play side by side with other children, but to connect with them on some fundamental level, sensing that they are to be trusted, that they enjoy spending time with him, and that he, in turn, looks forward to hanging out with them. Among that group of kids, there may be one with whom he feels most comfortable, and their playdates can foster a friendship that strengthens over time. There are no assurances, of course, but the future bodes well for most children on the spectrum as long as they receive intervention early and intensively, and you're there to support them along the way.

Does my child know I love him?

This is one of the most heart-wrenching questions parents we've interviewed ever shared with us, and for good reason. As parents, we want to know that our children understand how important they are to us. When we feel we're unable to reach them, we feel hopeless and saddened that they feel bereft and helpless when we can't find a way around their isolation. Science may not be able to detect with any certainty just how much autistic children comprehend their significance in their parents' lives, but measurable results aren't everything. If you've been your child's advocate all along, and you've loved him and showered him with as much affection as he will allow and accept (many autistic kids can't tolerate hugs), you can be sure that, somehow, he realizes you love him. He may not understand the complexity and depth of your love, but he can surely discern that you're the grown-up who's always by his side, rooting for him and taking him to meet all the helpful doctors and therapists he sees. He knows that you're the one who's there when he needs guidance, who's willing to lend a hand when he seems confused or angry or overwhelmed, and who applauds his victories, large and small. Those are acts of love, and love has its own language, one that few of us can break down. Love has a way of cutting through even the foggiest of emotional roads, somehow finding its destination time and again. Love your child and trust that he gets the message. He may not be able to reciprocate in the traditional way, but you are making a difference in his life. Even though he may not be able to confirm this to you right now, he grasps this on a very basic level.

Will my child become like the autistic adults I've seen in movies?

It's difficult to chart the course of autism definitively for all children, but if yours is receiving help and is enrolled in an appropriate educational environment—one that meets his developmental needs and pushes him to challenge himself—it's unlikely that he'll end up resembling the catatonic stereotypes portrayed on television and in movies. That's why it's so important to make sure he gets the help he needs *now,* and that his intervention programs evolve as he evolves, so that he'll continue to improve over time.

Will he be able to protect himself from unscrupulous people who may want to take advantage of his disorder?

Much depends on your child's developmental level and on what you've taught him thus far about the subject of bullies. Although we'd like to think that the world is generally benign and safe, there are unscrupulous and cruel people out there who seem to enjoy preying on the vulnerable. Because of his autism, your child can, unfortunately, become a target. Social stories (see chapter 5) may come in handy when it's time for you to discuss with him what to do when a person displays aggression toward him. The visual approach of social stories will allow you to illustrate "aggressive" versus "friendly" behavior, and what he can do to steer clear of the former.

You will have to be as specific with him as possible. Individuals on the spectrum have a hard time reading between the lines and deciphering such complex human behaviors as deception and betrayal. Faced with a bully who appears to be friendly but engages in rude behavior toward him, your child may not be able to tell "good" from "bad." That's why it's important that you keep track of those he befriends and vet them for him. You need to trust that he can form friendships on his own, especially as he gets older, but there's nothing wrong with looking out for his best interests. Over time and with practice and luck, he'll hone his skill at telling friends from enemies.

Will my child be able to hold down a regular job?

It's possible that your child will be gainfully employed as an adult, especially if he's high-functioning. Also, jobs that have specific duties outlined and that don't require intensive interaction with colleagues may work well for him. For example, if he's gifted at Web design, he may do well creating sites for clients as long as he doesn't have to recruit and manage them from day to day. It's helpful that the autism community has begun focusing on generating opportunities for autistic individuals by training them while they're still in school for various vocations and occupations. And thanks to the Americans with Disabilities Act, their rights are protected when it comes to job opportunities. If they're qualified and can perform their task, employers are not allowed to discriminate against them simply because they have the disorder. Now, whether companies are actively putting the ADA into practice is hard to police, but suffice it to say that if your child is able to perform a job, he should be able to seek employment in that particular field and be considered for the position, regardless of his autism.

Can my child live on his own when he grows up?

Very possibly. It's hard to know just how far your child's interventions and therapies will take him, but there's a very good chance that he'll be able to live independently when he's older, as long as he isn't severely impaired. (If this is the case, a number of residential treatment centers may assist your child once he reaches adulthood. Contact the local chapter of Autism Society of America for information about finding the appropriate community for your child.)

Temple Grandin, a scientist, college professor, and one of the most public faces of autism, has found a way to cope with the disorder into adulthood. She has harnessed it in such a way as to find a fulfilling career, live on her own, and inspire parents and children every day. As one of the foremost experts on autism, she is a tireless advocate who's continually promoting the need for research. Not everyone who's autistic can be a Temple Grandin, but many individuals who receive intensive therapies now may be able to become a vibrant part of their community.

Who will take care of my child when I'm no longer around?

This is a question that all parents face, and it's good that you're asking it now, as it's one that requires a great deal of planning on your end. Because your child leans on you a little more (perhaps a lot more) than most kids, you need to prepare for your future as well as his. While parents of typical children may be able to take some things for granted because their kids have fewer physical and cognitive challenges to face, they do, at some point, wonder in general terms whether their children will be all right. They also have to make provisions for the future to ensure that their kids are properly taken care of when the time comes. The main difference for parents of autistic children is that you may have to be extremely specific in your planning, and will have to put down in writing every minute detail.

Be sure you have a will in place that carefully outlines what will happen to your child should you or your partner pass away, and remember to update it as he gets older. Determine which relatives or friends you'd feel most comfortable making his guardian should the unthinkable happen and you and your partner die or become incapacitated. Make sure you discuss your plans with that designated person so he or she isn't surprised when the time comes. Pick someone who you know has a solid rapport with your child, and who cares for him almost as deeply as you do. If you can, start saving for his future now by putting aside money in a trust or savings account. A financial advisor at a local bank or brokerage firm can help you get started on this financial road.

If you have considerable assets, you may also want to consult an estate lawyer, who can help you plan for the needs of your child and the necessary transfer of assets when you pass away. A special-needs trust may be the best strategy for you, but discuss it first with your financial advisor and lawyer, as there are numerous and complicated tax advantages and disadvantages involved.

If your income is limited, your child may qualify for social security, either now or when he turns eighteen. Contact your local social security office to get more information on who qualifies and how to apply.

This question, however, speaks to a larger fear: that your child will be as dependent on you when he's an adult as he appears to be now. Although we can't predict that he'll grow out of the spectrum completely or be so high-functioning that he barely registers on the spectrum, there's every reason to hope that he stands a good chance of being able to take care of himself. By laying the foundation now and ensuring that he's receiving the proper treatments and education, you're paving the way for his future. Trust that it'll be bright and beautiful, if not exactly what you hoped it would be before you discovered he had autism.

Will my child ever fall in love and have children?

It's hard to predict this. Most parents, whether their children have developmental problems or not, wonder at one point or another if their kids will love and be loved. Love is the single most fundamental emotion, and we want nothing else but to know that our children will have a bright future in which they will make a profound connection with someone else and build a life and family together.

Clichéd as it may sound, love has no boundaries. It reaches beyond race, class, language, age, physical appearance, and abilities and has been known to put even the most unlikely individuals together. If your child has been able to interact with others, and the nature of his relationships is rich and deep, he may be able to sustain a long-term relationship with someone else and even have children. But his and his beloved's journey may not be smooth sailing all the way, as he'll likely continue to struggle with handling and deciphering emotions and communication issues. Nothing's impossible, however, and love has a way of trumping even the most vexing of problems.

Can my child have a life that is rewarding and joyful?

Yes, but it's important to ask yourself whose definition of "rewarding and joyful" you're using to describe the kind of life your child will be able to lead. If you're going by the traditional measures society seems to have right now (whether or not you agree that these measures are correct), your child may not pass the test. For example, some people will say that a rewarding life can be measured only by the ability to earn lots of money, own a house and a number of cars, and have children.

But if by "rewarding and joyful" you mean simply that he enjoys his life and has people who care for him, then you're already halfway there. For one thing, he has you and your partner and the rest of your family cheering him on. Plus, if he has a solid IEP or IFSP in place and continues to receive medical, emotional, and educational support from his extensive list of caregivers, therapists, doctors, teachers, and friends, then he'll continue to fashion a wonderful life. Like any typical child, he'll forge his own path and make headway into his grand future, one triumph at a time.

Resources

ALTERNATIVE THERAPEUTIC RESOURCES

American Hippotherapy Association
Coordinates healthcare providers who support equine movement for treatment purposes.
AHA Inc.
5001 Woodside Road
Woodside, CA 94062
888-851-4592
www.americanhippotherapyassociation.org
E-mail: info@americanhippotherapyassociation.org

American Music Therapy Association (AMTA)
A national organization devoted to increasing public awareness of the benefits of music therapy, and providing access to music therapy resources.
8455 Colesville Road, Suite 1000
Silver Spring, MD 20910
301-589-3300; fax: 301-589-5175
www.musictherapy.org

Great Strides Therapy
A hippotherapy resource owned and run by occupational therapist Elizabeth Sang.
14089 Scio Church Road
Chelsea, MI 48118
734-475-4304
www.greatstridestherapy.com

"Martial Arts and Physical Therapy: Exploring the Connections"
An article, posted on the American Physical Therapy Association's Web site, from the May 1, 2002, issue of *Physical Therapy Magazine* that defines the importance and value of martial arts therapy in individuals with disabilities.
www.apta.org/PTmagazine/Current_Issue?&id[1]=22828#24162

Music Therapy and Autism

From the Wings Learning Center, Intervention Resources section, an article entitled "Music Therapy and Autism in the Special Education Setting" shows how music therapy helps to develop communication skills, promote sensory engagement, and strengthen fine and gross motor function in autistic individuals.

Wings Learning Center
49 N. San Mateo Drive
San Mateo, CA 94401
650-342-8753; fax: 650-342-8763
www.wingslearningcenter.org/resources_4/music431.html

"Music Therapy and Language for the Autistic Child"

An article, posted on the Center for Autism's Web site, by Myra J. Staum, Ph.D., RMT-BC, Director and Professor of Music Therapy, Willamette University, Salem, Oregon, showing how music therapy leads to eye contact and development of speech in autistic individuals.

www.autism.org/music.html

North American Riding for the Handicapped Association (NARHA)

A nonprofit organization that illustrates the benefits of interactions with horses for individuals with special needs.

P.O. Box 33150
Denver, CO 80233
800-369-RIDE; fax: 303-252-4610
www.narha.org

United States Martial Arts Association

A nonprofit martial arts corporation, founded by O'Sensei Phil Porter, whose goal is to offer service and guidance to all martial artists. Included in the association's Web site is an easy-to-use international locator directory, helpful when researching martial arts organizations and martial arts therapy programs in your area.

916-727-1486; fax: 916-727-7236
www.mararts.org/index.shtml

Unlocking Physical Capabilities

The Web site of Martial Arts Therapy provides valuable insight on the benefits of martial arts for individuals with special needs.

Martial Arts Therapy

7800 W. Sharpe Road

Fowlerville, MI 48836

248-969-3705 or 517-223-7449

www.martialarts-therapy.com/index.html

EDUCATIONAL RESOURCES FOR HOME AND SCHOOL

Citizen's Alliance to Uphold Special Education (CAUSE)

A Michigan-based organization that provides important information, for those in and outside of Michigan, on special education and the laws governing it.

6412 Centurion Drive, #130

Lansing, MI 48917

517-886-9167 or 800-221-9105

www.causeonline.org

Hanen Center

A training resource that has been promoted by school districts and speech therapists and is easily applied in the home setting. Two of the center's guides, *It Takes Two to Talk* and *More than Words,* work on creating improved communication with your special-needs child.

1075 Bay Street, Suite 515

Toronto, ON M5S 2B1

Canada

416-921-1073; fax: 416-921-1225

www.hanen.org

Homeschooling Children Who "Aut" to be Home

Exploring everything about autism and homeschooling an autistic individual, from ABA to TEACCH, this site provides a tremendous amount of support and information from networks of homeschoolers.

www.home.earthlink.net/~tammyglaser798/authome.html

IDEA 97 (Individuals with Disabilities Education Act)

A United States Department of Education site providing information about IDEA, its amendments, applications, and resources.

U.S. Department of Education
400 Maryland Avenue, SW
Washington, DC 20202
800-USA-LEARN; TTY: 800-437-0833; fax: 202-401-0689
www.ed.gov/offices/OSERS/Policy/IDEA/index.html

Office of Special Education and Rehabilitative Services

United States Department of Education's program for providing funding and support to help state and local districts to improve leadership in special education.

Office of Special Education Programs
Office of Special Education and Rehabilitative Services
U.S. Department of Education
400 Maryland Avenue, SW
Washington, DC 20202
202-245-7531
www.ed.gov/about/offices/list/osers/osep/index.html?src=mr

Picture Exchange Communication System (PECS)

Picture cards designed to encourage autistic individuals to initiate conversation and allow for visual communication and prompts.

Pyramid Educational Consultants
226 West Park Place, Suite 1
Newark DE 19711
888-PECS-INC; fax: 302-368-2516
www.pecs.com

Residential Schools and Homes

Web site providing links to residential schools and homes for children and adults with autism and special needs.

www.members.tripod.com/trainland/residential.htm

Social Stories—The Gray Center for Social Learning and Understanding

A social story is a tool that describes an event, reason, place, cause, or action in a format that has significant meaning for autistic individuals.

The Gray Center for Social Learning and Understanding
2020 Raybrook SE, Suite 302
Grand Rapids, MI 49546
616-954-9747; fax: 616-954-9749
www.thegraycenter.org/Social_Stories.htm

State by State Contact Information for Department of Special Education

www.blind.net/bg330001.htm

TALC (The Advocacy and Learning Center)

Disseminates articles on its Web site that explain the IEP (Individualized Education Plan) process, parental preparation, IEP laws, and IEP resources.

C. M. Lowe
The Advocacy and Learning Center
3941 Park Drive, #20, PMB114
El Dorado Hills, CA 95762
Fax: 916-339-2475
www.pages.zdnet.com/ourorhskids/id23.html

TASH

An organization devoted to inclusion for individuals with disabilities.
29 West Susquehanna Avenue, Suite 210
Baltimore, MD 21204
Phone: 410-828-8274
www.tash.org

TEACCH (Treatment and Education of Autistic and related Communication handicapped CHildren)

A statewide program in North Carolina that provides families of autistic children with diagnostic, intervention, educational, and therapeutic services. TEACCH trains others around the world to use an individualized approach to autism, emphasizing individual assessment and planning for those on the spectrum.

Division TEACCH Association

CB#7180

100 Renee Lynne Court

University of North Carolina at Chapel Hill

Chapel Hill, NC 27599-7180

919-966-2174; fax: 919-966-4127

www.teacch.com

"Teaching Autistic Children Who Want to be Home"

An article by Tammy Glaser from *Home Education Magazine,* posted on a site that provides the whos, whats, whys, and hows for homeschooling a child with autism spectrum disorder.

www.homeschoolzone.com/add/autism.htm

Untangle Autism

An IEP center focusing on Individualized Education Plans for autistic individuals; a helpful database provides a multitude of examples of IEPs.

www.untangleautism.org/iep.htm

EVALUATION TOOLS AND DIAGNOSTIC RESOURCES

"Autism Related Disorders in *DSM–IV*"

An article written by Meredyth Goldberg Edelson, Ph.D., of the Department of Psychology at Willamette University in Salem, Oregon, outlining the diagnostic criteria used to identify varied facets of autism spectrum disorder as defined by the *Diagnostic and Statistical Manual of Mental Disorders–IV.*

Center for the Study of Autism
P.O. Box 4538
Salem, OR 97302
www.autism.org/dsm.html

First Signs: Screening Guidelines

An organization and Web site for pediatricians introducing early intervention guidelines for autism.

First Signs, Inc.
P.O. Box 358
Merrimac, MA 01860
978-346-4380; fax: 978-346-4638
www.firstsigns.org/screening/guidelines.htm

Is This Your Child?

A Canadian Web site promoting early diagnosis and intervention services for children with autism.

P.O. Box 1098
Burlington, ON L7R 4R8
Canada
www.autismcanada.org/pdfs/IsThisYourChild.pdf

The PDD Assessment Scale / Screening Questionnaire

A screening tool to show a possible diagnosis of PDD (Pervasive Developmental Disorders).

www.childbrain.com/pddassess.html

Reinforcement Unlimited

A clinic focusing on behavioral disorders, which provides evaluation and assessments that lead to devising an appropriate educational and interventional plan. They also sponsor training workshops for parents, educators, therapists, administrative staff, and medical professionals.

Robert W. Montgomery, Ph.D., BCBA
P.O. Box 1572
Woodstock, GA 30188
404-368-9100; fax: 770-516-4191
www.behavior-consultant.com

Understanding Autism Symptoms
From WebMD Health, a medical Web site that provides an outline of the symptoms of autism.

www.my.webmd.com/content/article/9/1680_54885?src= Inktomi&condition=Health%20Topics%20A-Z

FAMILY AND SOCIAL RESOURCES

Autism Friendly
Created by the father of an autistic child, this Web site identifies businesses (such as restaurants and shops) throughout the United States, sorted by zip code, that parents consider "autistic friendly." The site is updated by friends and family of autistic individuals.
www.autismfriendly.com

The Children Who Live with the Children of Autism
A Web resource to help parents understand the feelings and concerns of the nonautistic children in their families.

www.adamspublications.com/sibling.htm

National Respite Locator Service
Provides definition of respite care, a state-by-state locator, and respite camp contacts for children with special needs.

800 Eastowne Drive, Suite 105

Chapel Hill, NC 27514

919-490-5577; fax: 919-490-4905

www.respitelocator.org

Respite Care
Sometimes, those living with or caring for an individual with a chronic condition need time away from him or her to deal with their own care or the care of other family members. This site provides definition and careful introspection regarding respite care and resources about respite care organizations.

www.autism-pdd.net/respite.html

Sibling Support

A Web site created by the sister of a man with autism, providing support and education to siblings of autistic individuals.

www.siblingsofautism.com

The Sibling Support Project of the ARC of the United States

A Web site based on the belief that disabilities affect all members of a family, and providing support, resources, and information to siblings of children with special needs.

1010 Wayne Avenue, Suite 650

Silver Spring, MD 20910

301-565-5469; fax: 301-565-3843

www.thearc.org/siblingsupport

Special Needs Children Network

For families of children with special needs, discussing everything from social issues to relationship dilemmas.

www.specialneedschildrennetwork.com

Special Needs Family Resource Center

A Web site focused on the concerns of families with a member who has special needs, including autism.

514 South 4th Street

Philadelphia, PA 19147

215-592-1333; fax: 267-200-0806

www.specialfamilies.com

We the Siblings

Created by a teenager whose brother is autistic, this Web site provides support, friendship, and understanding to siblings of children with special needs.

www.angelfire.com/bc/autism

GENERAL AUTISM RESOURCES

Autistic Child Caution Signs
Web site that gives advice and helpful suggestions on how to obtain an "autism caution" sign for your neighborhood.

www.autisminmichigan.homestead.com/AutisticChildNeighborhood Sign.html

Autistic Continuum Connections, Education, and Support
A Web site created by autistic adults providing general information regarding ASD.

www.access.autistics.org

Autism One
A parent-created nonprofit organization focused on advocacy, education, and fundraising.

www.autismone.org

Autism Today
This organization's Web site provides resources for families and professionals dealing with autistic spectrum disorders.

2016 Sherwood Drive, Suite 3

Sherwood Park, AL T8A 3X3

Canada

780-482-1555; fax: 780-452-1098

U.S. Office:

1426 Harvard Avenue

Seattle, WA 98124

866-9AUTISM

www.autismtoday.com

Families for Early Autism Treatment (FEAT)
Based in California, this organization has chapters in many states and Canadian provinces, and provides resources on autism.

www.feat.org

Health Cyclopedia and Mental Health Disorders

This Web site is an encyclopedic guide to mental health disorders including diagnostic, treatment, prevention, and general information

www.healthcyclopedia.com/mental-health/disorders.html

NIMH Autism Spectrum Disorders (Pervasive Developmental Disorders)

The National Institute of Mental Health's site on autism includes information on history, symptoms, diagnosis, and treatment aid.

National Institute of Mental Health (NIMH)

Office of Communications

6001 Executive Boulevard, Room 8184, MSC 9663

Bethesda, MD 20892-9663

301-443-4513 or 866-615-6464; TTY: 301-443-8431;

fax: 301-443-4279

www.nimh.nih.gov/publicat/autism.cfm

Pervasive Developmental Disorders

Provides general information on PDDs.

P.O. Box 1492

Washington, DC 20013

800-695-0285; fax: 202-884-8441

www.nichcy.org/pubs/factshe/fs20txt.htm

Tony Attwood

Australian Web site run by a psychologist and autism expert, which examines issues and resources related to Asperger's Syndrome.

The Asperger's Syndrome Clinic

P.O. Box 224

Petrie

Queensland 4502

Australia

61 7 3285 7888

www.tonyattwood.com.au

University of Michigan Autism and Communication Disorders Center (UMACC)

Provides diagnostic, intervention, and educational services to assist the individual with autism and the community. The center's Web site provides resources about autism spectrum disorder.

UMACC
University of Michigan
1111 East Catherine Street
Ann Arbor, MI 48109-2054
734-936-8600
www.umaccweb.com

INTERVENTION RESOURCES

The Abilities Center

Provides information on therapeutic and intervention services and product resources.

5600 W. Maple Road, Suite A-100
West Bloomfield, MI 48322
248-855-0030
www.abilitiescenter.com

Center for the Study of Autism

A clearinghouse for information regarding autistic interventions.

P.O. Box 4538
Salem, OR 97302
www.autism.org

GFCF Diet Web site

Devoted to introducing and providing support and resources for autistic individuals and their families on the gluten-free, casein-free diet.

www.gfcfdiet.com

Dr. Barry Prizant

Prizant and other clinicians are the innovators of the SCERTS (Social Communication, Emotional Regulation, Transactional Support) model of intervention services.

Barry M. Prizant, Ph.D., CCC-SLP
2024 Broad Street
Cranston, RI 02905
401-467-7008
www.barryprizant.com

RDI (Relationship Development Intervention)

The Web site of Dr. Steve Gutstein introduces his treatment program. RDI is an intervention for individuals with autism spectrum disorder that helps them to become flexible and creative thinkers and aids them in communication and connectivity to others.

4120 Bellaire Boulevard
Houston, TX 77025
713-838-1362; fax: 713-838-1447
www.connectionscenter.com

Son-Rise Program

Sponsored by the Autism Treatment Center of America, the program trains parents to create a home-based program for the child with autism.

Autism Treatment Center of America
2080 S. Undermountain Road
Sheffield, MA 01257
413-229-2100 or 877-SONRISE; fax: 413-229-3202
www.son-rise.org

LEGAL RESOURCES

Americans with Disabilities Act (ADA)

The United States Department of Justice's official Web site for ADA provides information about the ADA and its applications and purpose.

U.S. Department of Justice

950 Pennsylvania Avenue, NW
Civil Rights Division
Disability Rights Section – NYAV
Washington, DC 20530
800–514–0301; TTY: 800–514–0383; fax: 202–307–1198
www.ada.gov

ADA (Americans with Disabilities Act) Investigative Agencies

This Web site supplies contact information for specific agencies with whom individuals can file complaints if they feel their rights have been violated in the following areas: education, employment, government, housing, health, and human services.
www.ada.gov/investag.htm

The National Autistic Society

A British organization that advocates and assists individuals with autism.
The National Autistic Society
393 City Road
London EC1V 1NG
United Kingdom
44 (0)20 7833 2299; fax: 44 (0)20 7833 9666
www.nas.org.uk

Partners in Policymaking

A program that trains individuals with special needs and their parents to become advocates for those with disabilities.
www.partnersinpolicymaking.com

Unlocking Autism

A group that educates the public about autism, provides funding for research and assistance, and supports autistic individuals and their families.
9463 Florida Boulevard, Suite D
Walker, LA 70785
225–665–7270
www.unlockingautism.org

Wrightslaw

Web site for expert information on special-education law, IEP (Individualized Education Plan) guidance, and advocacy for children with special needs.

www.wrightslaw.com

MEDICAL RESOURCES

American Academy of Pediatrics

A resource Web site dedicated to children's health issues.
American Academy of Pediatrics National Headquarters
141 Northwest Point Boulevard
Elk Grove, IL 60007-1098
847-434-4000; fax: 847-434-8000
www.aap.org

Apraxia Kids

Information and resources for individuals dealing with speech apraxia.
www.apraxia-kids.org/index.html

Autism Biomedical Information Network (ABINet)

Provides biomedical information on autism.
ABINet
P.O. Box 1393
Highland Park, IL 60035
www.autism-biomed.org

Autism Research Institute

Nonprofit organization that provides research and shares research on the causes of autism, prevention, diagnosis, and treatment.
4182 Adams Avenue
San Diego, CA 92116
www.autism.com/ari

Brain Wonders

Information on brain development from conception to age three.

202-638-1144

www.zerotothree.org/brainwonders

Centers for Disease Control and Prevention (CDC)

The search engine on the Centers' Web site links to many valuable autistic resources and information on autism research and resources.

www.cdc.gov

The following page of the CDC Web site focuses on the National Center on Birth Defects and Developmental Disabilities and has an information center highlighting autism:

www.cdc.gov/ncbddd/dd/ddautism.htm

The following page lists links on vaccine and autism theories:

www. cdc.gov/nip/vacsafe/concerns/autism/default.htm

Childbrain.com

From Dr. Rami Grossman of the Child Neurology and Developmental Center, this site provides information on the latest technologies and concerns surrounding many neurological conditions, including autistic spectrum disorders.

Child Neurology and Developmental Center

6 Tuxedo Avenue

New Hyde Park, NY 11040

516-739-7799; fax: 516-739-7768

www.childbrain.com

or

146-01 45th Avenue, Suite 401

Flushing, NY 11355

www.childbrain.com/index.shtml

Clinical Trials.Gov

A Web site created by the National Library of Medicine and serviced by the National Institutes of Health, providing up-to-date information on human clinical research. Much information is provided on autism spectrum disorders, including research trials involving Fragile X.

Reference and Customer Services
National Library of Medicine
8600 Rockville Pike
Bethesda, MD 20894
888-346-3656
www.clinicaltrials.gov/ct/
gui;jsessionid=DC7F42FC9B2AB16490961685D0ADED46

Cure Autism Now (CAN)
Created by a group of parents and clinicians, CAN promotes biomedical research and education on autism.
5455 Wilshire Boulevard, Suite 715
Los Angeles, CA 90036
323-549-0500 or 888-8AUTISM; fax: 323-549-0547
www.cureautismnow.org/index.jsp

FRAXA Research Foundation
Disseminates information on Fragile X.
FRAXA Research Foundation
45 Pleasant Street
Newburyport, MA 01950
978-462-1866; fax: 978-463-9985
www.fraxa.org

Genetics Home Reference Page
A Web site providing guidance on genetic conditions such as Rett
Syndrome.
www.ghr.nlm.nih.gov/ghr/
;jsessionid=9A7530563D3364C242954BD647B9C551

The Mayo Clinic
A highly respected not-for-profit institute of health and research based
in Rochester, Minnesota.
200 First Street SW
Rochester, MN 55905
507-284-2511
www.mayoclinic.org

National Alliance for Autism Research (NAAR)

An organization whose goal is to promote scientific and biomedical autism research.

99 Wall Street, Research Park

Princeton, NJ 08540

888-777-NAAR; fax: 609-430-9163

www.naar.org/naar.asp

National Institute of Child Health and Human Development

The institute's Web site posts an in-depth article entitled "Autism and Genes": www.nichd.nih.gov/publications/pubs/autismandgenes.pdf. The site discusses possible causes of autism and examines ongoing research in an article entitled "The Collaborative Programs of Excellence in Autism (CPEAs)": www.nichd.nih.gov/autism/dpea.cfm.

National Institute of Child Health and Human Development

P.O. Box 3006

Rockville, MD 20847

800-370-2943; fax: 301-496-7101

National Vaccine Information Center

A nonprofit organization working to change the vaccination protocols in place in the United States.

421-E Church Street

Vienna, VA 22180

703-938-DPT3

www.909shot.com

National Vaccine Injury Compensation Program

A program from the United States Department of Health and Human Services providing information for those who feel they or a family member were injured through an inoculation.

National Vaccine Injury Compensation Program

Parklawn Building

5600 Fishers Lane, Room 16C-17

Rockville, MD 20857

800-338-2382

www.hrsa.gov/osp/vicp/fact_sheet.htm

The Seaver Center for Autism Research and Treatment

A treatment center that does pioneering research into the biological causes of autism and similar disorders. Projects include neuroimaging and autoimmune studies.

Mount Sinai School of Medicine
Department of Psychiatry
Box 1230
One Gustave L. Levy Place
New York, NY 10029
www.mssm.edu/psychiatry/autism

University of Michigan Health System: "Your Child" Website

An informative Web site that provides guidance on child development and behavior and includes a special area on autism.

www.med.umich.edu/1libr/yourchild

Zero to Three

A nonprofit national organization that promotes health research for children of infant and toddler age.

www.zerotothree.org

NEWSLETTER RESOURCES

Bridges 4 Kids

An "all-for-one" Web site featuring legal, health, social, and educational resources for families of children with special needs. The organization also has a newsletter to which you can subscribe.

www.bridges4kids.org

The Schafer Autism Report

A newsletter focusing on all matters related to autism.
9629 Old Placerville Road
Sacramento, CA 95827
www.sarnet.org

ON-LINE AUTISM SUPPORT GROUPS

Autism Awareness Action Yahoo Group
An international group for sharing autism information.
health.groups.yahoo.com/group/autism-awareness-action

Autism Spectrum Yahoo Group
An informal support group.
health.groups.yahoo.com/group/Autism-Spectrum

Children with Autism Yahoo Group
An international advocacy group.
groups.yahoo.com/group/children_with_autism

Everyday Miracles
A parent-led support, resource, and advocacy group that hosts live on-line presentations from autism experts and support meetings in the state of Michigan, and also distributes a hard copy newsletter.
health.groups.yahoo.com/group/EverydayMiraclesAutism

Everything Autism Yahoo Group
A great place to discuss anything and everything about the world of autism.
groups.yahoo.com/group/EVERYTHING-AUTISM

Parents-to-Parents Autism Group
This network of parent support and parent information exchange on autism also features open online chat sessions.
health.groups.yahoo.com/group/P2ParentsChat

(To join the above autism groups or to find other autism on-line groups, visit the Yahoo group site at groups.yahoo.com)

Asperger's Listserv

A moderated e-mail listserv for individuals interested in receiving information about the disorder.

To join, e-mail: listserv@maelstrom.stjohns.edu and put in the subject line: subscribe asperger.

Autism List: St. John's University

A parent-run e-mail list based in Australia.

http://hunter.apana.org.au/~cas/autismlist/autintro.html

Babycenter.com: Parenting a Child with Autism Spectrum Disorder

A bulletin board for moms and dads of children on the spectrum who want to share strategies and offer support.

http://bbs.babycenter.com/board/toddler/toddlerdevelopment/
1143871

GFCF Diet Community Bulletin Board

An online community of parents and children who are on the gluten-free, casein-free diet.

www.gfcfdiet.com/communitybulletinboard.htm

iVillage.com/Parentsoup: Autism

Message boards and information that cater to families with special-needs children and offer them support and guidance.

www.parentsoup.com

Urbanbaby.com

A Web site with local bulletin boards for parents of children in more than half a dozen cities with special needs (most of them dealing with autism).

www.urbanbaby.com

PRODUCTS FOR AUTISTIC CHILDREN

Hanging Sky Chairs
Chairs that can be hung inside or out, and provide comfort, relaxation, and vestibular input for children with ASD.

800-759-8759; fax: 303-938-9735

www.skychairs.com

National Autism Registry Cards
A Web site from which cards can be ordered for use in public places, to declare that your child has autism and cannot tolerate long lines, and to explain autism and its consequential behaviors.

www.dimensionsspeech.com/autism-registry.htm

The PLAY Project (Play and Language for Autistic Youngsters) CD-ROM
A CD-ROM to train parents, medical professionals, therapists, and educators in the Floortime Model created by Dr. Stanley Greenspan and personified by Dr. Richard Solomon's PLAY Project.

www.playproject.org/cdrom.htm

The Self Esteem Shop
A store that provides toys and books promoting confidence-building in children and adults with special needs.

32839 Woodward Avenue

Royal Oak, MI 48073

248-549-9900 or 800-251-8336; fax: 248-549-0442

www.selfesteemshop.com

Sensory Resources
An online shop for sensory resources and products.

2500 Chandler Avenue, Suite 3

Las Vegas, NV 89120-4064

702-433-0404 or 888-357-5867; fax: 702-891-8899

www.sensoryresources.com

Southpaw Enterprises
Distributor of sensory integration therapy products.
P.O. Box 1047
Dayton, OH 45401
937-252-8502 or 800-228-1698
www.southpawenterprises.com

Visual Strategies
Information, resources, and products for visual support services.
QuirkRoberts Publishing
P.O. Box 71
Troy, MI 48099-0071
248-879-2598; fax: 248-879-2599
www.UseVisualStrategies.com

PRODUCT RESOURCES

Autism Children's Books
A Web site listing books that explain autism for both children with autism and their peers.
Future Horizons, Inc.
721 West Abram Street
Arlington, TX 76013
800-489-0727; fax: 817-277-2270
www.autism-childrensbooks.com

Flaghouse Catalog
Their "special populations" catalog offers a variety of books on various interventions, from speech and sensory to occupational and physical therapies.
U.S.A.: 201-288-7600 or 800-793-7900
Canada: 416-495-8262 or 800-265-6900
Mexico: 5567-6484
www.flaghouse.com

**Books for and about autistic individuals (fiction/biography/
autobiography):**

Grandin, Temple. *Thinking in Pictures: And Other Reports from My Life
with Autism.* New York: Random House, 1996.

A memoir by one of the foremost experts on autism that provides
a fascinating peek into the mind of an individual who's on the spectrum herself.

Grandin, Temple, and Margaret Scariano. *Emergence: Labeled Autistic.*
New York: Warner Books, 1996.

Grandin discusses her diagnosis and how she overcame what was
once thought of as a permanently debilitating disorder.

Haddon, Mark. *The Curious Incident of the Dog in the Night-Time.* New
York: Doubleday, 2003.

An award-winning, critically acclaimed novel told from the perspective of Christopher Boone, a boy with Asperger's.

Holliday Willey, Lianne, and Tony Attwood. *Pretending to be Normal:
Living with Asperger's Syndrome.* London: Taylor & Francis Group, 1995.

A mother whose daughter also has Asperger's charts her efforts to
manage her and her child's condition in this engrossing account.

Hornby, Nick, editor. *Speaking with the Angel.* New York: Riverhead,
2001.

A short-story anthology edited by celebrated British writer Hornby,
whose autistic son authored one of the stories included. Also features
stories by Zadie Smith, Dave Eggers, and Helen Fielding. Proceeds
benefit charities devoted to autism causes worldwide.

LaSalle, Barbara. *Finding Ben.* New York: McGraw-Hill, 2003.

A kindergarten teacher explores the issues and struggles her family
has faced since her son, Ben, was found to be on the spectrum.

Paradiz, Valerie. *Elijah's Cup: A Family's Journey into the Community and Culture of High-Functioning Autism and Asperger's Syndrome.* New York: Free Press, 2002.

A memoir by a Bard College professor about how her family's existence was turned upside down when her child was diagnosed with Asperger's Syndrome.

Seroussi, Karen. *Unraveling the Mystery of Autism and Pervasive Developmental Disorder: A Mother's Story of Research and Recovery.* New York: Broadway Books, 2002.

A mother details her son's personal experience with autism, from diagnosis at 19 months to finding success with various interventions.

Stacey, Patricia. *The Boy Who Loved Windows: Opening the Heart and Mind of a Child Threatened with Autism.* Cambridge: Da Capo Press, 2003.

A searing and heartbreakingly honest memoir by a mother of an autistic child about her efforts to seek appropriate treatment for her son.

Williams, Donna. *Somebody, Somewhere: Breaking Free from the World of Autism.* California: Three Rivers Press, 1995.

An Australian artist exposes her struggles with autism and multiple personalities.

SUPPORT RESOURCES

ARC of the United States
National organization that promotes the need for the integration of all special-needs individuals into their own community.
1010 Wayne Avenue, Suite 650
Silver Spring, MD 20910
301-565-5469; fax: 301-565-3843
www.thearc.org

Autism Society of America

Organization providing support, services, and information for individuals with autism and their family, friends, teachers, and healthcare providers.

For a state-by-state chapter listing of the Autism Society of America:
www.autism-society.org/site/PageServer?pagename=chaptermap
For general Autism Society of America information and resources:
www.autism-society.org
7901 Woodmont Avenue, Suite 300
Bethesda, MD 20814-3067
301-657-0881 or 800-3AUTISM

Benevolent and Protective Order of Elks of the USA

A group with chapters in local communities, providing assistance and support to children with special needs.

BPO Elks of the USA
2750 N. Lakeview Avenue
Chicago, IL 60614-1889
773-775-4400; fax: 773-775-4790
www.elks.org

Center for Autism and Related Disabilities (CARD)

An organization that assists individuals with autism and similar disabilities.

CARD/Gainesville
P.O. Box 100234
Gainesville FL 32610-0234
352-846-2761 or 800-754-5891; fax: 352-846-0941
www.card.ufl.edu

Disabilities Today

A Web site that offers current information for those with disabilities and educates the public about individuals with special needs.

www.disabilitiestoday.com

Doug Flutie Jr. Foundation for Autism

An organization established by football star Doug Flutie in honor of his son, Doug Flutie Jr., who has ASD, this foundation raises funds for autism research and provides financial support to economically disadvantaged families.

P.O. Box 767
Framingham, MA 01701
866-3AUTISM
www.dougflutiejrfoundation.org
E-mail: info@dougflutiejrfoundation.org

Fighting Autism

A group that advocates quality-of-life improvements for children with ASD through research, education, advocacy, and treatment.

351 Ivy Drive
Gibsonia, PA 15044
412-641-7383
www.fightingautism.org

4 Paws for Ability

A group that advocates the use of service dogs to help autistic individuals.
253 Dayton Avenue
Xenia, OH 45385
937-374-0385
www.4pawsforability.org/autismdogs.htm

National Service Dogs Training Center

A service organization whose members train dogs to assist autistic individuals and their families.

1251 Puddicombe Road
New Hamburg, ON N0B 2G0
Canada
519-662-4223; fax: 519-662-4697
www.nsd.on.ca

Parents of Autistic Children of Massachusetts (POAC)

Provides education and information to parents of children with autism and the professionals who work with individuals on the spectrum.

P.O. Box 583
Woburn, MA 01801
978-455-2160
www.poac.net

University of Michigan Dance Marathon

The University of Michigan Dance Marathon is one of several organizations at universities throughout the United States that raise funds for programs designed for children with special needs. It hosts parties, activities, and outings throughout the school year for special-needs children, their siblings, and their families.

www.umdm.org

THERAPEUTIC RESOURCES

ABA Resources for Recovery from Autism/PDD/Hyperlexia

In-depth information on ABA compiled by a father of a child with autism.

http://rsaffran.tripod.com/aba.html

Association for Metroarea Autistic Children, Inc.

One of the leading centers for applied behavior therapy (ABA), AMAC provides diagnostic services, runs a summer camp, and a program for autistic adults.

25 West 17th Street
New York, NY 10011
www.amac.org

Bright Tots Speech and Language Resource Guide

Information on how speech therapy can be beneficial to a child with autism.

917-647-6252
www.brighttots.com/speechtherapy.html

Cambridge Center for Behavioral Studies

An organization devoted to the application of behavioral studies to alleviate human suffering, offering on its Web site information on behavioral intervention and specifically applied behavioral analysis for those with autism.

Cambridge Center for Behavioral Studies Publication Office
336 Baker Avenue
Concord, MA 01742-2107
978-369-CCBS; fax: 978-369-8584
www.behavior.org/autism/index. cfm?page=http%3A/
www.behavior.org/autism/autism_costbenefit.cfm

Cleveland Clinic's Center for Autism

Diagnostic, intervention, and educational assistance provided for children on the autistic spectrum.

Cleveland Clinic Children's Hospital for Rehabilitation
2801 Martin Luther King Jr. Drive
Cleveland, OH 44104
216-721-5400
www.clevelandclinic.org/childrensrehab/programs/autism

Easter Seals

An organization offering affordable services, such as speech and occupational therapy, for children and adults with special needs.

230 West Monroe Street, Suite 1800
Chicago, IL 60606
312-726-6200 or 800-221-6827; TTY: 312-726-4258;
fax: 312-726-1494
www.easterseals.com

Floortime Foundation

The Web site of Dr. Stanley Greenspan and his interventive program of Floortime based on his DIR (Developmental Individual-Difference Relationship–Based) model.

410-486-1251
www.floortime.org

Help for Kids Speech

A nationwide program, sponsored by the Scottish Rite Foundation of
Florida, helping families of children with communication disorders and
assisting them in finding therapeutical assistance.

www.helpforkidspeech.org

Hope Center for Autistic Children

A center at Beaumont Hospital in Michigan that provides ABA training for parents of children with autism who attend sessions with their children. General information on ABA is provided on the center's Web site.

248-691-4744

www.beaumonthospitals.com/pls/portal30/cportal30.webpage?l_
recent=center_hope#

Lovaas Institute for Early Intervention (LIFE)

An early intervention center promoting the UCLA Model of Applied
Behavioral Analysis to teach children with autism in a comprehensive
setting.

11500 West Olympic Boulevard, Suite 460

Los Angeles, CA 90064

310-914-5433; fax: 310-914-5463

www.lovaas.com

The PLAY Project (Play and Language for Autistic Youngsters)

Created by Dr. Richard Solomon, PLAY is a model based on Floortime. The project's Web site includes information on Floortime, the PLAY
Project, research, conference events, and articles, and how to purchase a
training CD-ROM.

www.playproject.org

Sensory Integration International (SSI)

Information regarding sensory integration therapy and the pioneering
work of Dr. A. Jean Ayres in this field.

P.O. Box 5339

Torrance, CA 90510-5339

310-787-8805; fax: 310-787-8130

www.home.earthlink.net/~sensoryint/

Selected References

Americans with Disabilities Act (ADA). United States Department of Justice. www. ada/gov.

American Academy of Pediatrics—Immunization Initiatives. "The Pediatrician's Role in the Diagnosis and Management of Autistic Spectrum Disorder in Children." Committee on Children with Disabilities (2001). http://search.aap.org/aap/CISPframe.html?url=http://www.cispimmunize.org/fam/mmr/a_report2.html.

Association in Manhattan for Autistic Children, Inc. (AMAC). School Observation. May 25, 2004.

"Autism: New Findings on Social Interaction Deficits in Autism and Schizophrenia." *Drug Week,* December 2003.

Autism Research Foundation and LADDERS Clinic. "Current Trends in Autism." Conference. Newton, MA, October 24, 25, 26, 2003.

Autism Society of America. "ASA Statement on May 2004 IOM Report on Vaccines and Autism." www.autism-society.org/site/PageServer?pagename=mmrvaccine.

——. "Biomedical and Dietary Treatments." http://www.autism-society.org/site/PageServer?pagename=BiomedicalDietaryTreatments.

Autism Today. "Genetic Factors in Autism." www.autismtoday.com/articles/Genetic_Factors_in_Autism.htm.

Band, Eve B., and Emily Hecht. *Autism Through a Sister's Eyes.* Arlington, Texas: Future Horizons, 2001.

Baron-Cohen, Simon. *The Essential Difference: The Truth about the Male and Female Brain.* New York: Basic Books, 2003.

Baron-Cohen, Simon, J. Allen, and C. Gilbert. "Can Autism Be Detected at 18 Months: The Needle, the Haystack, and the CHAT." *British Journal of Psychology* 161 (1992): 839–843.

BarryPrizant.com. "About Barry M. Prizant, Ph.D, CCC-SLP." www.murphyandmurphy. com/barryprizant/barryprizant/about.cfm.

——. "The SCERTS Model." www.murphyandmurphy.com/barryprizant/scerts/model. cfm.

Bertrand, J., A. Mars, C. Boyle, F. Bove, M. Yeargin-Allsopp, P. Decouflé. "Prevalence of Autism in a United States Population: The Brick Township, New Jersey, Investigation." *Pediatrics* 108, no. 6 (2001).

Blausten, Frederica. Interview by authors. New York City, 25 May 2004.

Boblitt, Pat. Phone interview by authors. Sebastol, California. July 2004.

Bondy, Andrew S., and Lori A. Frost. "The Picture Exchange Communication System." *Focus on Autistic Behavior* (August 1994).

——. "The Picture Exchange Communication System." Reprinted from *The Advocate.* www.pecs.com/asaPEC3panel.html.

Brasic, James Robert. "Pervasive Developmental Disorders and Autism." Carol Dianne Berkowitz et al., eds. *E-Medicine: Instant Access to the Minds of Medicine at Johns Hopkins University School of Medicine* (November 3, 2003) www.emedicine.com/ped/topic180. htm.

Campbell, Carol Ann. "Researchers Challenging Assumptions About Autism." *Newshouse News Service,* January 3, 2003.

——. "Study Yields Promising Ties Between Gene and Autism." *Newshouse News Service,* April 26, 2004.

Centers for Disease Control. "Autism Information Center." National Center on Birth Defects and Developmental Disabilities. www.cdc.gov/ncbddd/dd/aic/about/default.htm.

——. "Institutes of Medicine Reports: Immunization Safety Review" www.cdc.gov/nip/news/iom-main.htm.

——. "Vaccines and Autism Theory." www.cdc.gov/nip/vacsafe/concerns/autism/default.htm

"Children's Hospital of Philadelphia: Parents of Children with Autism Turn to Medical Alternatives." *Biotech Week,* January 28, 2004.

Cleveland Clinic Center for Autism, *A New Beginning: Center for Autism Offers Hope to Children and Parents.* Pamphlet.

ClinicalTrials.gov. "Autistic Disorder." http://clinicaltrials.gov/ct/gui/action/FindCondition? ui=D001321&recruiting=true

College of Optometrists and Vision Development. "Vision and Autism." www.covd.org.

Committee on Children with Disabilities. "The Pediatrician's Role in the Diagnosis and Management of Autistic Spectrum Disorder in Children." *Pediatrics* 107, no. 5 (May 2001): e85. http://pediatrics.aappublications.org/cgi/content/full/107/5/e85.

Conan, Neil. "Effects of Autism on Families." *National Public Radio: Talk of the Nation,* January 21, 2003.

Cook, Edwin H. Jr., Bennett L. Leventhal, and David H. Ledbetter. "The Role of Genetics in the Diagnosis of Autistic Disorder." www.agre.org/reference/fullarticles/draft. html.

Critchley, Hugo D., et al. "The Functional Neuroanatomy of Social Behavior: Changes in Cerebral Blood Flow When People with Autistic Disorder Process Facial Expressions." *Brain: Journal of Neurology,* 123, no. 11 (November 2000): 42–52.

Cunningham, Eleese, and Wendy Marcason. "Question of the Month: Is There Any Research to Support a Gluten- and Casein-Free Diet for a Child That Is Diagnosed . . ." *Journal of the American Dietetic Association* 101, no. 2 (February 1, 2001): 222.

"Dealing with the Public." Electronic mail responses from Betty Carlson, Carol Curotto, Kitty Bradford, Kristi Walter, Miranda Turner, and Sherry Franklin, April and May 2004.

DeFrancesco, Laura. "Autism on the Rise: Multi-Disciplinary Efforts Aim at Finding the Biological Basis for a Complex Disease." *The Scientist* 15, no. 10 (May 14, 2001): 16.

Division TEACCH–The University of North Carolina at Chapel Hill. "What is TEACCH?" www.teacch.com.

Dooley, Pamela, Felicia Wilczenski, and Christopher Torem. "Using an Activity Schedule to Smooth School Transitions." *Journal of Positive Behavior Interventions* 3, no. 1 (January 2001): 57.

Dunlap, Glen, Lee Kern, and Jonathan Worchester. "ABA and Academic Instruction." *Focus on Autism and Other Developmental Disabilities* 16, no. 2 (Summer 2001): 129–136.

Durand, V. Mark. "New Directions in Educational Programming for Students with Autism." Dianne Berkell Zager, ed. *Autism: Identification, Education, and Treatment.* Mahwah, New Jersey: Lawrence Erlbaum Associates, 1999. 323–343.

Edwards, Bob, with Jon Hamilton. "Effort to Get First Accurate Count of Children with Autism." *National Public Radio: Morning Edition,* January 26, 2004.

"Family and Social Dynamics Inquiry." Electronic mail responses from Ginnene Stone, Kelly Zigulis, Kris Oudsema, and Sharon Cohen, July 2004.

Gerstein, Leonore. Phone interview by authors. July 2004.

Glover, Laura. Phone interview by authors. July 2004.

Goin, Robin P., and Barbara J. Meyers. "Characteristics of Infantile Autism: Moving Toward Earlier Detection." *Focus on Autism and Other Developmental Disabilities* 19, no. 1 (April 1, 2004): 5.

Goode, Erica. "Autism Cases Up: Cause Is Unclear." *The New York Times,* January 26, 2004.

———. "Lifting the Veils of Autism, One by One." *The New York Times,* February 24, 2004.

Gordon, C.T. "New CDC Report Shows Prevalence of Autism Is Higher." *Narrative Journal of the National Alliance for Autism Research* (Spring 2003): 11.

———. "Science and Research: Pharmacological Treatment Options for Autism." *Narrative Journal of the National Alliance for Autism Research* (Spring 2003): 8–10.

Gormley, Mike. "Playmates for Nicholas." *Charlotte Observer,* July 21, 2004.

Grandin, Temple. "Evaluating the Effects of Medication." Center for the Study of Autism. www.autism.org/temple/meds.html.

———. *Thinking in Pictures: And Other Reports from My Life with Autism.* New York: Random House, 1996.

The Gray Center. "ASD." www.thegraycenter.org/autism_spectrum_disorders.htm.

Greenspan, Stanley I., and Serena Weider. "Basic Principles of Floortime." Richard Solomon, ed. *The PLAY Project Manual,* 2000.

———. "The Infancy and Childhood Training Course." Conference. Tyson's Corner, Virginia, April 23, 24, 25, 26, 2004.

Greenspan, Stanley, Serena Weider, and Robin Simons. *The Child with Special Needs.* New York: Perseus Books, 1998.

Gupta, Sanjay. "An In-Depth Look at Autism." *CNN Sunday Morning Show: Weekend House Call* (September 7, 2003).

Hart, Nigel. "With Autism I'm a Different Person Inside. It's as Though I'm Looking at Life Out of a Window: Charlie Agar Aims to Train, Educate, and Make People More Understanding of Her Disability." *Coventry Evening Telegraph,* May 15, 2002, 8–9.

Hatch-Rasmussen, Cindy. "Sensory Integration." Center for the Study of Autism. www.autism.org/si.html.

Hays, Kathleen, Valerie Morris, and Stephanie Elam. "The Rise in Autism: Increase in Cases Tremendous." *CNNFN The Flip Side,* April 1, 2004.

Hill, Whitley. "Pushing Play." *Medicine at Michigan* 4, no. 3 (Fall 2002): 28–33.

Hite, Wendy. Autism and education inquiry electronic mail responses, June 2004. "The Autism Information Center" and "About Autism." www.cdc.gov/ncbddd/dd/aic/about/default.htm./

Hoekman, Laurel A. "Sensory Integration." The Gray Center. www.thegraycenter.org/sensory_integration.htm.

Hurd, Lyle. "Restoring Health and Detoxifying Your Baby," *Total Health,* September/October 2002.

IDEA Practices. "Laws and Regulations." www.ideapractices.org/law/index.php.

Jacobson, John W., James A. Mulick, and Gina Green. "EIBI Saves up to $2,500,000: Summary—Cost Benefits Estimates for Early Intensive Behavioral Intervention for Young Children with Autism." *Behavioral Interventions* 13 (1998): 201–226. www.behavior.org/autism/index.cfm?page=http%3A//www.behavior.org/autism/autism_costbenefit.cfm.

James, R. B. "PET Scanning in Autism Spectrum Disorders." Dean Wong, Aylin Eroglu, Sydney Louis, et al., eds. *E-Medicine: Instant Access to the Minds of Medicine at Johns Hopkins University School of Medicine* (August 22, 2003). www.emedicine.com.

Jensen, Vanessa K., and Leslie V. Sinclair. "Treatment of Autism in Young Children: Behavioral Intervention and Applied Behavioral Analysis." *INF Young Children* 14, no. 4 (2002): 42–52.

Kaufman, Curtis, et al. "Fluvoxamine Treatment of a Child with Severe PDD: A Single Case Study." *Psychiatry* 64, no. 3 (October 1, 2001): 268.

Kimball, Jonathan W. "Behavior-Analytic Instruction for Children with Autism: Philosophy Matters." *Focus on Autism and Other Disabilities* 17, no. 2 (Summer 2002), p. 66.

Koegel, Robert L., Jennifer B. Symon, and Lynn Kern Koegel. "Parent Education for Families of Children with Autism Living in Geographically Distant Areas." *Journal of Positive Behavior Interventions* 4, no. 2 (April 2002): 88.

Koenig, Kathleen, and Lawrence Scahill. "Assessment of Children with Pervasive Developmental Disorders." *Journal of Child and Adolescent Psychiatric Nursing* 14, no. 4 (October 2001): 159.

Kunzig, Robert. "Autism: What's Sex." *Psychology Today,* January/February 2004.

Laeburn, Paul. "Understanding the Biological Causes of Autism." *National Public Radio: Talk of the Nation/Science Friday,* January 24, 2003.

Lears, Laurie, and Karen Ritz. *Ian's Walk: A Story about Autism.* Morton Grove, Illinois: Albert Whitman and Company, 2003.

Lindsay, Ronald L., and Michael G. Aman. "Pharmacologic Therapies Aid Treatment for Autism." *Pediatric Annals,* 32, no. 10 (October 1, 2003): 671.

"Lovaas: The Man Behind the Theory—The Creator of ABA." What You Need to Know About. http://autism.about.com/library/weekly/aa092000a.htm.

Mestal, Rosie. "Autism Drug Fails Latest Clinical Trial: Despite Disappointing Test Results Some Advocates of Secretin Therapy Hold Out Hope." *Los Angeles Times,* January 12, 2004.

National Academies, News Office. "Early Intervention Is Key to Educating Children with Autism." The National Academies. June 13, 2001. www4.nationalacademies.org/news.nsf/0a254cd9b53e0bc585256777004e74d3/67fb3bf368f0c9a985256ca70072dc45?OpenDocument.

National Alliance for Autism Research. "What is Autism?—History." www.naar.org/aboutaut/whatis_hist.htm.

National Immunization Program. "Vaccines and Autism: An Institute of Medicine (IOM) Report: Immunization Safety Review: Vaccines and Autism (May 2004)." CDC. http://www.cdc.gov/nip/news/iom-thim5-18-04.htm.

——. "Autism and Genes." National Institutes of Health. http://www.nichd.nih.gov/publications/pubs/autismandgenes.pdf.

Newman, Bobby, et al. *Graduated Applied Behavioral Analysis—AMAC (Association in Manhattan for Autistic Children, Inc.).* New York: Dove and Orca, 2002.

Newnham, David. "Autism Features and Art." Supplement to *The New York Times,* no. 4408, 15.

Olney, Marjorie. "Working with Autism and Other Social-Communication Disorders." *Journal of Rehabilitation* (October-December 2000).

Painter, Kim. "Science Getting to the Root of Autism." *USA Today,* January 12, 2004.

Parent Focus Group on Autism. January 29, 2004.

"Perseveration." Electronic mail inquiry responses from Betsy Carlson, Carol D. Curotto, Dan Rakowski, Kim Lewis, Kristi Walter, Laura Suzanne, Mary Beth Langan, Terri Shock, Virginia Dyke, and other parents who wish to remain anonymous, March 2004.

Peterson, Iver. "High Rewards and High Costs as State Draws Autistic Pupils." *The New York Times,* May 26, 2000.

"Picture Exchange Communication System." Pyramid Educational Consultants, Inc. www.pecs.com/page5.html.

The PLAY Project (Play and Language for Autistic Youngsters). "Level II Workshop." Canton, Michigan, April 10, 2004.

Pollack, Andrew. "Secretin Does Not Aid Autism: Trial—No More Effective Than Placebo." *National Post (Canada),* January 8, 2004, sec. Body and Health.

——. "Trials and Parents' Hopes for Autism Drug." *The New York Times,* January 6, 2004.

Powers, Michael D., ed. *Children with Autism: A Parent's Guide,* 2nd ed. Bethesda: Woodbine House, 2000.

Prizant, Barry, et al. "The SCERTS Model: A Transactional, Family-Centered Approach to Enhancing Communication and Socioemotional Abilities of Children with Autism Spectrum Disorder." *Infants and Young Children* 16, no. 4 (2003): 296.

Rapin, Isabelle. "Autism." *New England Journal of Medicine* 337, no. 2 (July 10, 1997): 97.

———. Electronic mail messages regarding perseveration, March 2004.

Robinsong, Sayulita. Phone interview by authors. August 2004.

Rock, Andrea. "Toxic Tipping Point." *Mother Jones* (March/April 2004). www.mojones.com/news/feature/2004/03/02_354.html.

Romanczyk, Raymond G., et al. "Research in Autism: Myths, Controversies, and Perspectives." Dianne Berkell Zager, ed. *Autism: Identification, Education, and Treatment.* Mahwah, New Jersey: Lawrence Erlbaum Associates, 1999. 23–61.

Seipel, Tracy, and Marian Liu. "As Autism Cases Increase, Research and Treatment Improves." *San Jose Mercury News,* June 18, 2002.

Sheehan, Susan. "The Autism Fight." *The New Yorker* (December 1, 2003).

Simpson, Richard L. "ABA and Students with Autism Spectrum Disorder: Issue and Considerations for Effective Practice." *Focus on Autism and Other Developmental Disabilities* 16, no. 2 (Summer 2001): 68–71.

———. "Individualized Educational Programs for Students with Autism: Including Parents in the Process." *Focus on Autistic Behavior* (October 1995).

Solomon, Richard. "Intensive Interventions for Young Children with Autism Spectrum Disorders." Richard Solomon, ed. *The PLAY Project Manual.*

———. Interview by authors. Ann Arbor, Michigan. July 2004.

Stacey, Patricia. "Floortime." *The Atlantic Monthly* (January/February 2003): 127–134.

———. *The Boy Who Loved Windows: Opening the Heart and Mind of a Child Threatened with Autism.* Cambridge, Massachusetts: Da Capo Press, 2003.

Symons, Jennifer B. "Parent Education for Autism: Issues in Providing Services at a Distance." *Journal of Positive Behavior Interventions* 3, no. 3 (July 2001): 160.

Taylor, Brent, et al. "Measles, Mumps, and Rubella Vaccination and Bowel Problems or Developmental Regression in Children with Autism . . ." *British Medical Journal (International Edition)* 324, no. 7334 (February 16, 2002): 393.

Thomas, Carol. Phone interview by authors. Summer 2003.

Thompson, Mary. *Andy and His Yellow Frisbee.* Bethesda: Woodbine House, 1996.

Thrower, David, et al. "Correspondence." *The Lancet* 363, no. 9408 (February 14, 2004): 567.

Tsai, Luke Y. "Medical Treatment in Austism." Dianne Berkell Zager, ed. *Autism: Identification, Education, and Treatment.* Mahwah, New Jersey: Lawrence Erlbaum Associates, 1999. 199–257.

Tyrell, Fiona. "One Man's Story Reveals the Dangers of Not Fully Understanding Autism." *The Irish Times,* April 6, 2004.

U.S. Congress. House of Representatives. House Appropriations Committee. Testimony by Robert L. Beck, President and CEO of Autism Society of America. *Fiscal 2005 Appropriations: Labor, HHS, Education.* April 27, 2004.

———. House Government Reform Committee. Testimony by Bernard Rimland of the Autism Research Institute. *The Future Challenges of Autism.* November 19, 2003.

———. Senate. House Government Reform Committee. *U.S. Representative Dan Burton of Indiana Holds Hearings on Vaccines and Autism.* December 10, 2002.

Voigt, Robert G., et al. "Early Pediatric Neurodevelopment Profile of Children with Autistic Spectrum Disorders." *Clinical Pediatrics* 39, no. 11 (November 2000): 663.

Volkmar, Fred R., and David Pauls. "Autism." *The Lancet* 362 (October 2003): 1133.

Yell, Mitchell, et al. "Developing Legally Correct and Educationally Appropriate Programs for Students with Autism Spectrum Disorders." *Focus on Autism and Other Developmental Disabilities* 18, no. 3 (October 2003): 182.

Zager, Dianne Berkell, ed. *Autism: Identification, Education, and Treatment.* Mahwah, New Jersey: Lawrence Erlbaum Associates, 1999.

Index